T0348709

Colonoscopic Polypectomy

Editor

DOUGLAS K. REX

GASTROINTESTINAL ENDOSCOPY
CLINICS OF NORTH AMERICA

www.giendo.theclinics.com

Consulting Editor
CHARLES J. LIGHTDALE

October 2019 • Volume 29 • Number 4

ELSEVIER

1600 John F. Kennedy Boulevard • Suite 1800 • Philadelphia, Pennsylvania, 19103-2899

http://www.theclinics.com

GASTROINTESTINAL ENDOSCOPY CLINICS OF NORTH AMERICA Volume 29, Number 4
October 2019 ISSN 1052-5157, ISBN-13: 978-0-323-70866-1

Editor: Kerry Holland
Developmental Editor: Donald Mumford

Gastrointestinal Endoscopy Clinics of North America (ISSN 1052-5157) is published quarterly by Elsevier Inc., 360 Park Avenue South, New York, NY 10010-1710. Months of issue are January, April, July, and October. Business and Editorial Offices: 1600 John F. Kennedy Blvd., Suite 1800, Philadelphia, PA, 19103-2899. Periodicals postage paid at New York, NY and additional mailing offices. Subscription prices are $359.00 per year for US individuals, $624.00 per year for US institutions, $100.00 per year for US students and residents, $399.00 per year for Canadian individuals, $737.00 per year for Canadian institutions, $476.00 per year for international individuals, $737.00 per year for international institutions, and $245.00 per year for Canadian and international students/residents. To receive student/resident rate, orders must be accompanied by name of affiliated institution, date of term, and the *signature* of program/residency coordinator on institution letterhead. Orders will be billed at individual rate until proof of status is received. Foreign air speed delivery is included in all *Clinics* subscription prices. All prices are subject to change without notice. **POSTMASTER:** Send address change to *Gastrointestinal Endoscopy Clinics of North America*, Elsevier Health Sciences Division, Subscription Customer Service, 3251 Riverport Lane, Maryland Heights, MO 63043. **Customer Service: 1-800-654-2452 (US). From outside the United States, call 1-314-447-8871. Fax: 1-314-447-8029. E-mail: JournalsCustomerService-usa@elsevier.com (for print support) or JournalsOnlineSupport-usa@elsevier.com (for online support)**.

Reprints. For copies of 100 or more, of articles in this publication, please contact the Commercial Reprints Department, Elsevier Inc., 360 Park Avenue South, New York, NY 10010-1710. Tel. 212-633-3874; Fax: 212-633-3820; E-mail: reprints@elsevier.com.

Gastrointestinal Endoscopy Clinics of North America is covered in *Excerpta Medica, MEDLINE/PubMed (Index Medicus), and MEDLINE/MEDLARS.*

Contributors

CONSULTING EDITOR

CHARLES J. LIGHTDALE, MD
Professor of Medicine, Division of Digestive and Liver Diseases, Columbia University Medical Center, New York, New York, USA

EDITOR

DOUGLAS K. REX, MD, MACP, MACG, FASGE, AGAF
Distinguished Professor of Medicine, Division of Gastroenterology and Hepatology, Indiana University School of Medicine, Chancellors Professor, Indiana University-Purdue University Indianapolis, Director of Endoscopy, Indiana University Hospital, Indianapolis, Indiana, USA

AUTHORS

RAVISHANKAR ASOKKUMAR, MD
Consultant, Department of Gastroenterology and Hepatology, Singapore General Hospital, Singapore, Singapore

KENNETH BINMOELLER, MD
Director of Endoscopy, Interventional Endoscopy Services, California Pacific Medical Center, San Francisco, California, USA

MICHAEL J. BOURKE, MBBS, FRACP
Director of Endoscopy, Department of Gastroenterology and Hepatology, Endoscopy Unit, Westmead Hospital, Professor of Medicine, Westmead Clinical School, University of Sydney, Sydney, New South Wales, Australia

ARSHISH DUA, MD
Gastroenterology Fellow, Division of Gastroenterology, Loyola University Medical Center, Stritch School of Medicine, Maywood, Illinois, USA

ANNA M. DULOY, MD
Therapeutic Endoscopy Fellow, Division of Gastroenterology and Hepatology, University of Colorado Anschutz Medical Center, Aurora, Colorado, USA

NORIO FUKAMI, MD, AGAF, FACG, FASGE
Director of Advanced Endoscopy, Division of Gastroenterology and Hepatology, Professor, Mayo Clinic College of Medicine and Science, Mayo Clinic, Scottsdale, Arizona, USA

NEIL GUPTA, MD, MPH, FASGE
Regional Director, Digestive Health Program, Associate Professor of Medicine, Division of Gastroenterology, Stritch School of Medicine, Director of Interventional Endoscopy, Loyola University Medical Center, Maywood, Illinois, USA

DAVID G. HEWETT, MBBS, MSc, PhD, FRACP
Faculty of Medicine, The University of Queensland, Department of Gastroenterology, Queen Elizabeth II Jubilee Hospital, Brisbane Colonoscopy, Brisbane, Queensland, Australia

BILEL JIDEH, BMedSci, MBBS, FRACP
Advanced Endoscopy Fellow, Department of Gastroenterology and Hepatology, Endoscopy Unit, Westmead Hospital, Clinical Lecturer, Westmead Clinical School, University of Sydney, Sydney, New South Wales, Australia

CHARLES J. KAHI, MD, MS, FACP, FACG, AGAF, FASGE
Professor of Clinical Medicine, Indiana University School of Medicine; Gastroenterology Section Chief, Roudebush VA Medical Center, Indianapolis, Indiana, USA

TONYA KALTENBACH, MD, MS
Associate Professor of Medicine, Department of Gastroenterology, Veterans Affairs Medical Center, Department of Medicine, University of California, San Francisco, California, USA; Advanced Gastrointestinal Endoscopy, Mountain View, California, USA

RAJESH N. KESWANI, MD, MS
Associate Professor of Medicine, Department of Gastroenterology and Hepatology, Northwestern University, Chicago, Illinois, USA

AMMAR O. KHEIR, MBBS, MRCP, FRACP
Faculty of Medicine, The University of Queensland, Department of Gastroenterology, Queen Elizabeth II Jubilee Hospital, Brisbane, Queensland, Australia; Endoscopy, QEII Hospital, Queensland, Australia; Digestive Disease Institute, Cleveland Clinic Abu Dhabi, Abu Dhabi, UAE

BRIAN LIEM, DO
Associate Program Director, Gastroenterology Fellowship, Assistant Professor of Medicine, Division of Gastroenterology, Stritch School of Medicine, Loyola University Medical Center, Maywood, Illinois, USA

CARMEL MALVAR, BA
Department of Gastroenterology, Veterans Affairs Medical Center, Department of Medicine, University of California, San Francisco, California, USA

ANDREW NETT, MD
Interventional Endoscopy Services, California Pacific Medical Center, San Francisco, California, USA

TIFFANY NGUYEN-VU, BA
Department of Gastroenterology, Veterans Affairs Medical Center, Department of Medicine, University of California, San Francisco, California, USA

GOTTUMUKKALA SUBBA RAJU, MD, FASGE
John Stroehlein Distinguished Professor, Department of Gastroenterology, Hepatology and Nutrition, The University of Texas MD Anderson Cancer Center, Houston, Texas, USA

DOUGLAS K. REX, MD, MACP, MACG, FASGE, AGAF
Distinguished Professor of Medicine, Division of Gastroenterology and Hepatology, Indiana University School of Medicine, Chancellors Professor, Indiana University-Purdue University Indianapolis, Director of Endoscopy, Indiana University Hospital, Indianapolis, Indiana, USA

SILVIA SANDULEANU, MD, PhD
Associate Professor of Medicine, Division of Gastroenterology and Hepatology, Maastricht University Medical Center, Maastricht, The Netherlands

AMRITA SETHI, MD
Associate Professor of Medicine, Director of Interventional Endoscopy, Division of Digestive and Liver Disease, Columbia University Medical Center – NewYork-Presbyterian Hospital, New York, New York, USA

ROY SOETIKNO, MD, MS, MSM
Professor of Medicine, Advanced Gastrointestinal Endoscopy, Mountain View, California, USA; University of Indonesia, Kampus Baru UI Depok, Jawa Barat, Jakarta, Indonesia

NICHOLAS J. TUTTICCI, MBBS, FRACP
Faculty of Medicine, The University of Queensland, Department of Gastroenterology, Queen Elizabeth II Jubilee Hospital, Brisbane, Queensland, Australia; Endoscopy, QEII Hospital, Queensland, Australia

KAVEL VISRODIA, MD
Fellow in Interventional Endoscopy, Division of Digestive and Liver Disease, Columbia University Medical Center – NewYork-Presbyterian Hospital, New York, New York, USA

Contents

Colonoscopic polypectomy is fundamental to effective prevention of colorectal cancer. Polypectomy reduces colorectal cancer incidence and mortality by altering the natural history and progression of precancerous precursor polyps. Epidemiologic data from the United States, where colorectal cancer rates have been steadily declining in parallel with screening efforts, provide indisputable evidence about the effectiveness of polypectomy. Randomized controlled trials of fecal occult blood tests and flexible sigmoidoscopy, and observational colonoscopy studies, provide additional support. Longitudinal studies have shown variable levels of protection after polypectomy, highlighting the central importance of high quality and adequate surveillance of higher-risk patients.

 Video content accompanies this article at http://www.giendo. theclinics.com.

Ineffective polypectomy technique may lead to incomplete polyp resection, high complication rates, interval colorectal cancer, and costly referral to surgery. Despite its central importance to endoscopy, training in polypectomy is not standardized nor has the most effective training approach been defined. Polypectomy competence is rarely reported and quality metrics for this skill are lacking. Use of tools and measurements to assess polypectomy outcomes is low. There is a need for standardization of training and remediation in polypectomy; defining standards of competent polypectomy and how it is feasibly measured; and integration of polypectomy quality metrics into training programs and the accreditation process.

Diminutive colorectal lesions are polyps and flat lesions 1 to 5 mm in size, and small are 6 to 9 mm in size. The best resection method is the cold snare. Cold forceps are acceptable for 1- to 3-mm lesions, but should not be used to piecemeal polyps. Cold snaring has few complications and is more effective than cold forceps for 4- to 5-mm polyps and as effective and more efficient than hot snaring for 6- to 9-mm polyps.

poorly executed submucosal injection may increase the difficulty and risk of EMR. Underwater EMR (UEMR), an alternative resection method for colonic neoplasms, avoids the need for submucosal injections. In comparison with reported outcomes of EMR, UEMR achieves similar rates of complete resection with comparable safety, with lower rates of recurrence and fewer repeat procedures. UEMR also compares favorably with endoscopic submucosal dissection in terms of procedure time and rates of complete resection, recurrence, and complications.

Endoscopic resection for large colorectal lesion is effective and cost-saving than surgery. Piecemeal resections are often effective if applied meticulously but endoscopic submucosal dissection (ESD) allows meritorious removal of large lesions in one piece. For rectal lesions, transanal endoscopic microsurgery or transanal minimally invasive surgery offers more radical transmural resection but ESD is also effective for removal of complex rectal lesions. Surgical resection with lymph node dissection is the gold standard for invasive cancer; however, the management of low-risk early-stage colorectal cancer is worth debating. Treatment selection for large colorectal lesions is discussed based on lesion factor and treatment outcomes.

 Video content accompanies this article at http://www.giendo. theclinics.com.

Retrieval of lesions after endoscopic polypectomy enables histopathologic analysis and guides future surgical management and endoscopic surveillance intervals. Various techniques and devices have been described with distinct advantages and disadvantages to accomplish retrieval. Appropriate histopathologic analysis depends on lesion handling and preparation. How lesions are handled further depends on size, endoscopic appearance, and removal technique. Endoscopic marking or tattooing is a well-described process that uses dye mediums to leave longstanding marks in the colon. Techniques, dye mediums, and locations within the colon influence tattoo approach.

Large and complex colon polyps are frequently referred to surgery for fear of perforation that may need emergency surgery. During the last 15 years, advances in clip and suturing devices allowed us to close perforations and avoid surgery. In addition, we have made substantial progress in our understanding of the lesions at risk for either immediate or delayed perforation. This article focuses on the colonoscopic closure of resection defects and perforations and the prevention and treatment of colon perforations after endoscopic resection.

Nicholas J. Tutticci, Ammar O. Kheir, and David G. Hewett

Cold resection for small colonic polyps, and larger lesions, is being rapidly and widely adopted. Driven by an impressive safety and cost profile compared with conventional polypectomy, these advantages are offset by the limitations of smaller and shallower resection, and absent thermal effects that may permit persistence of residual neoplasia. To overcome this, optimal cold snare technique requires inclusion of a margin of normal mucosa and a piecemeal resection technique for larger polyps. This article examines the fundamentals of cold snare resection and evidence for its application, theorizes on limits to its application, and identifies areas for further research.

GASTROINTESTINAL ENDOSCOPY CLINICS OF NORTH AMERICA

FORTHCOMING ISSUES

January 2020
Endoscopic Closures
Roy Soetikno and Tonya Kaltenbach,
Editors

April 2020
Management of GERD
Kenneth J. Chang, *Editor*

July 2020
Colorectal Cancer Screening
Douglas K. Rex, *Editor*

RECENT ISSUES

July 2019
Inflammatory Bowel Disease
Simon Lichtiger, *Editor*

April 2019
The Endoscopic Hepatologist
Christopher J. DiMaio, *Editor*

January 2019
**Gastroparesis: Current Opinions and New
EndoscopicTherapies**
Qiang Cai, *Editor*

RELATED CLINICS SERIES

Gastroenterology Clinics
Clinics in Liver Disease

THE CLINICS ARE AVAILABLE ONLINE!
Access your subscription at:
www.theclinics.com

Foreword

Colonoscopic Polypectomy: Improved and New Methods

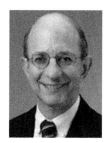

Charles J. Lightdale, MD
Consulting Editor

Once it became clear that most colorectal cancers developed from premalignant colon polyps, screening colonoscopy with removal of these polyps became the focus of colon cancer prevention with demonstrable effectiveness. The brilliant simplicity of the flexible cautery snare quickly became the standard method for polypectomy, and the use of partial colon resections to remove precancerous colon polyps plummeted. As colonoscopy evolved with an emphasis on higher detection of adenomas and identification of subtle flat colon lesions such as sessile serrated adenomas, the need for improved polypectomy techniques has become obvious. In addition, new methods, such as endoscopic mucosal resection (EMR), endoscopic submucosal dissection, and endoscopic full thickness resection, have been successfully applied in the colon and rectum.

This issue of *Gastrointestinal Endoscopy Clinics of North America* is devoted entirely to colonoscopic polypectomy. I am extremely pleased that the editor for this issue is Dr Douglas K. Rex, a world-renowned leader in the field. He has assembled an outstanding group of international expert authors to cover all the key aspects of modern colon polyp removal. The amount of detailed information provided in this single issue of *Gastrointestinal Endoscopy Clinics of North America* on the subject of colonoscopic polypectomy is extraordinary and unprecedented. Topics covered include a review of the evidence that polypectomy prevents cancer, how to assess polypectomy quality, how to teach polypectomy, and how to characterize flat and depressed colon lesions in planning resection. Techniques for removal of both small and large polyps are presented, and how to retrieve specimens and when and how to close postpolypectomy wall defects. The increasing use of noncautery "cold" resection is discussed as well as the innovative underwater EMR approach. This issue should be read in its entirety by every practicing colonoscopist, along with quality and endoscopy unit

Gastrointest Endoscopy Clin N Am 29 (2019) xiii–xiv
https://doi.org/10.1016/j.giec.2019.06.008
1052-5157/19/© 2019 Elsevier Inc. All rights reserved.

giendo.theclinics.com

directors. Don't miss this issue! It will bring you completely up-to-date and will almost certainly make you better at what you do.

Charles J. Lightdale, MD
Department of Medicine
Columbia University Medical Center
161 Fort Washington Avenue
New York, NY 10032, USA

E-mail address:
CJL18@columbia.edu

Preface

Colonoscopic Resection in Evolution

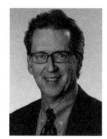

Douglas K. Rex, MD, MACP, MACG, FASGE, AGAF
Editor

Five decades have passed since the introduction of colonoscopy and the transformative development of the wire loop polypectomy snare by Shinya, Wolff, and Ichikawa in the United States and Deyhle in Europe. Remarkably, the wire snare remains the workhorse of everyday colonic resection. Despite this, very important changes in colonoscopic resection have appeared in the current century. First, colonoscopic resection has changed from an anecdotal practice in which colonoscopists largely used whatever techniques they acquired in training, with academic centers often using substantially different approaches based largely on tradition, into a clinical science. Michael Bourke and his consortium of Australian investigators with their work on endoscopic mucosal resection have been pivotal in this transformation to a scientific approach to resection. Other important and emerging trends include reliance on cold (without electrocautery) resection of small and some larger lesions, with the promise of reduced complications. The exciting development of underwater mucosal resection has been led by Ken Binmoeller. The emergence of endoscopic submucosal dissection for selected colorectal lesions has been slowed in the United States by several practical considerations, but is gaining traction. Very importantly, we now recognize that even basic colonoscopic resection skills vary by up to 3-fold between endoscopists in the same practice, and that detection and resection are 2 different endoscopic skills that have poor correlation with each other. Thus, we are on the threshold of extension of the colonoscopy quality movement from prioritizing detection-based indicators to include measurement of polypectomy skill.

This issue is stuffed with practical tips and explanations of modern colonoscopic resection methods. I am deeply indebted to the world class experts who have contributed to this issue and am confident that any colonoscopist can utilize these pages to

Gastrointest Endoscopy Clin N Am 29 (2019) xv–xvi
https://doi.org/10.1016/j.giec.2019.06.009
1052-5157/19/© 2019 Published by Elsevier Inc.

giendo.theclinics.com

become up-to-date on best practices of this critical procedure, one that saves thousands of lives around the world each year.

Douglas K. Rex, MD, MACP, MACG, FASGE, AGAF
Indiana University School of Medicine
Indiana University Hospital
550 North University Boulevard
Suite 4100
Indianapolis, IN 46202, USA

E-mail address:
drex@iu.eu

Reviewing the Evidence that Polypectomy Prevents Cancer

Charles J. Kahi, MD, MS

KEYWORDS

- Colorectal neoplasms • Polypectomy • Prevention • Colonoscopy

KEY POINTS

- The main effector of colorectal cancer prevention is polypectomy.
- Widespread polypectomy has been a major driver of declining colorectal cancer incidence and mortality in the United States.
- Evidence of the effectiveness of polypectomy is derived from epidemiologic data and from studies of the outcome of patients after fecal occult blood testing and after lower endoscopy.
- High quality polypectomy is central to effective colorectal cancer prevention.

INTRODUCTION

The concept of colorectal cancer (CRC) screening has transformed over the past few decades, with the realization that the benefit is primarily from prevention of cancer via detection and elimination of premalignant lesions and secondarily from detection of early curable-stage cancers. The amenability to primary prevention is a fundamental characteristic of CRC, which distinguishes it from other screenable cancers, where the focus is generally on secondary prevention via detection of early stage malignancy.[1] This paradigm originated in 1965 with Gilbertsen and colleagues,[2] who postulated that CRC could be prevented by polypectomy, and was later supported by the biologic framework of the Fearon-Vogelstein adenoma-carcinoma sequence.[3] It is now accepted that most CRCs develop within precursor adenomatous or serrated polyps and that interruption of the polyp-to-cancer sequence prevents the development of CRC. The effect of interrupting the progression to CRC on patient outcomes has been the subject of multiple investigations. Several observational studies have reported reduced CRC incidence and mortality after colonoscopy.[4–14] These studies were heterogeneous, however, and included patients with no findings and those with various

Disclosure statement: The author has nothing to disclose.
Indiana University School of Medicine, Roudebush VA Medical Center, 1481 West 10th Street, 111G, Indianapolis, IN 46202, USA
E-mail address: ckahi2@iu.edu

Gastrointest Endoscopy Clin N Am 29 (2019) 577–585
https://doi.org/10.1016/j.giec.2019.05.001
1052-5157/19/Published by Elsevier Inc.
giendo.theclinics.com

precursor polyp types and numbers. This heterogeneity affects the interpretability of the findings, because it is known from several negative colonoscopy studies[15–19] that patients without polyps are a lower-risk group among the broader average-risk population. It is important to understand these differences, because prevention of CRC by endoscopic procedures is not due to the identification of persons without polyps but rather to the detection and complete resection of polyps in patients with colorectal neoplasia. In other words, the main effector of CRC prevention is polypectomy.

There are currently no data from randomized controlled trials (RCTs) to determine the effect of polypectomy on CRC incidence and mortality. Isolating the effect of polypectomy would require a randomized design with a control group where polyps are left in situ without resection, which is neither a reasonable nor ethical consideration. There are 4 large ongoing RCTs[20–23] in Europe and the United States comparing colonoscopy to fecal immunochemical testing for CRC screening that could clarify the impact of polypectomy, but their results will not be available for years. Despite the lack of RCT-level data, the effectiveness of polypectomy to prevent CRC is indisputable. Proof of this assertion is derived from several lines of evidence, including epidemiologic data, RCTs of fecal occult blood tests (FOBTs) and flexible sigmoidoscopy, and observational colonoscopy studies.

EPIDEMIOLOGIC OBSERVATIONS

CRC is a worldwide scourge with globally increasing burden. The United States has been an epidemiologic exception, however, with steadily decreasing incidence rates since the 1980s[24] and long-term projections predicting declines through 2030.[25] There has been debate regarding the relative contribution of risk factor modification to the US CRC epidemiologic trends, because the declines began prior to the mass screening era.[26] It is impossible not to attribute a majority of the progress to awareness and compliance with screening, however, and attendant widespread removal of precancerous polyps: in the United States, CRC declines have been most noticeable in those 65 years and older and have accelerated for proximal colon cancer in the past decade,[24] observations that are likely driven by increased use of colonoscopy and polypectomy especially after screening colonoscopy became a Medicare benefit in 2001. The more recently noted increases in CRC incidence in persons less than 50 years old,[27] who are not routinely screened for CRC, provides an additional indirect argument that polypectomy is largely responsible for CRC decreases in screening-eligible age groups. That more colonoscopy and polypectomy could alter CRC epidemiology at the population level is supported by recent evidence from Germany, where CRC incidence and mortality have begun to decrease 10 years after colonoscopy was added to the German national cancer screening program.[28]

EVIDENCE FROM FECAL OCCULT BLOOD TEST STUDIES

RCTs have consistently shown that screening with FOBTs is associated with reductions in CRC mortality, ranging from 15% to 33%.[29–33] The FOBT is primarily a test for the detection of CRC, and it can be argued that the beneficial effect of FOBT-based screening strategies is derived from detection of early-stage cancers. Studies reporting the long-term outcomes of patients after FOBT screening suggest, however, that colonoscopy with polypectomy is a major contributor to the observed reductions in CRC mortality. The Minnesota Colon Cancer Control Study[34] randomized 46,551 participants to annual or biennial FOBT screening or usual care. Through 30 years of follow-up, screening was associated with lower CRC mortality with annual (relative risk [RR] 0.68; 95% CI, 0.56–0.82) and biennial screening (RR 0.78; 95% CI, 0.65–0.93) compared with usual care, whereas all-cause mortality was not significantly different. Importantly, the CRC mortality reduction of 32% at 30 years was sustained throughout the observation period and similar to estimates at earlier time points. If early detection of CRC was the primary mechanism by which FOBT screening led to decreased CRC mortality, the benefit would have been most apparent during the first few years of follow-up after removal of CRC cases from the cohort, then deteriorated over time. The lack of such an observation strongly suggests that in patients with positive FOBT, colonoscopy with polypectomy and subsequent colonoscopic surveillance are responsible for the sustained long-term reduction in CRC mortality. An earlier analysis of the Minnesota FOBT cohort attributed a 20% reduction in CRC incidence after 18 years to colonoscopy with resection of polyps.[35]

A more modest reduction in CRC mortality of 13% was reported after 20 years of follow-up of patients in the Nottingham FOBT RCT and no reduction in CRC incidence despite the removal of more than 600 large adenomas in the intervention arm.[36] The Nottingham and Minnesota trials, however, differed in key aspects, notably the use of nonrehydrated FOBT, leading to lower positivity and subsequent colonoscopy rates and lower participant compliance rates in the Nottingham RCT.

EVIDENCE FROM SIGMOIDOSCOPY STUDIES

The results of sigmoidoscopy-based screening have been extrapolated to colonoscopy because they both are structural examinations of the colon and utilize the same endoscopic technology. RCTs of screening sigmoidoscopy have reported significant reductions in CRC incidence and mortality, and meta-analyses have reported overall CRC mortality reductions of approximately 28%.[37,38]

The UK RCT[39] assessed more than 170,000 participants who were assigned to sigmoidoscopy or control groups, of which approximately 5% were referred to colonoscopy for large, histologically advanced, or multiple adenomas. In intention-to-treat analyses, after 11 years of follow-up, CRC incidence was reduced by 23% (hazard ratio [HR] 0.77; 95% CI, 0.70–0.84) and mortality by 31% (HR 0.69; 95% CI, 0.59–0.82) in the sigmoidoscopy group. After median follow-up of 17 years, CRC incidence and mortality reductions were 26% and 30%, respectively.[40] The Prostate, Lung, Colorectal and Ovarian (PLCO) cancer RCT[41] randomized 154,900 participants to screening sigmoidoscopy (repeated at 3 years or 5 years) or to usual care. After a median of 12 years, CRC incidence was reduced by 21%, and CRC mortality by 26%. It is, however, difficult to isolate the effect of polypectomy performed in the sigmoidoscopy RCTs and separate it from that of subsequent colonoscopies, because the trials used different polyp resection policies at the time of sigmoidoscopy and different colonoscopy referral strategies and colonoscopy utilization and contamination varied between studies. For example, in the PLCO trial, patients with polyps at sigmoidoscopy were advised to undergo colonoscopy with approximately 80% compliance rate; conversely, the contamination rates in the usual care arm were 26% for flexible sigmoidoscopy and 34% for colonoscopy.[41] A meta-analysis showed that colonoscopy was associated with a 40% to 60% lower risk of incident CRC and death from CRC than sigmoidoscopy, which was statistically significant only for deaths due to proximal cancer.[42] Additional insight can be derived from the outcome of patients with polyps at sigmoidoscopy after referral to colonoscopy, as reviewed in the following section.

EVIDENCE FROM COLONOSCOPY STUDIES

The first colonoscopy study to demonstrate unequivocally that polypectomy is a powerful tool to prevent CRC was the National Polyp Study (NPS)[43] in 1993, and has become the reference standard for subsequent polypectomy studies (**Table 1**). The NPS cohort included 1418 patients who underwent colonoscopy with resection of at least 1 adenoma and followed for a mean of 6 years. Five asymptomatic CRCs were detected during surveillance, corresponding to a 76% reduction in CRC compared with a Surveillance, Epidemiology, and End Results (SEER) reference group, and no CRC deaths occurred. The long-term NPS follow-up study[44] provides compelling proof of the effectiveness of polypectomy to prevent CRC: the cohort included 2602 patients with adenomas (including the 1418 who were randomized in the original NPS assessing surveillance intervals after colonoscopy) followed for up to 23 years after polypectomy. Compared with a SEER control population, CRC mortality was reduced by 53% (95% CI, 20%–74%), and the reduction for the first 10 years was similar to after 10 years of follow-up. In addition, CRC mortality was similar among adenoma patients compared with an internal control group with nonadenomatous polyps for the first 10 years after polypectomy (RR 1.2; 95% CI, 0.1–10.6).

An Italian observational prospective cohort study[45] of 1693 patients who underwent colonoscopic polypectomy of adenomas greater than or equal to 5 mm reported a 66% (95% CI, 37%–77%) CRC incidence reduction compared with the general Italian population. The Funen Adenoma Follow-up Study,[46] which assessed surveillance intervals in patients with adenomas, reported significant reductions in CRC incidence and mortality for up to 24 years after adenoma resection: compared with the Danish population, CRC incidence RR was 0.65 (95% CI, 0.43–0.95) and CRC death RR was 0.12 (95% CI, 0.03–0.36). Other adenoma cohort studies have shown less impressive reductions in CRC incidence after polypectomy. The Wheat Bran Fiber Trial[47] and Polyp Prevention Trial[48] assessed the effect of fiber to prevent adenoma recurrence after polypectomy, and both reported much higher CRC incidence rates compared with the NPS (2.2 vs 0.6 per 1000 patient-years). Another study[49] combined data from 3 adenoma chemoprevention RCTs, which assessed the effect of calcium, folic acid, antioxidants, and aspirin on recurrence rates of colorectal adenomas after colonoscopy and polypectomy. The overall incidence of CRC was 1.74 (95% CI, 1.05–2.72) per 1000 person-years of follow-up, compared with 0.6 and 0.4 in the NPS and Italian studies, respectively, and was not significantly different from expected

Table 1 Selected observational studies of colorectal cancer incidence and mortality after colonoscopic polypectomy			
Study	**N**	**Follow-up (y)**	**Colorectal Cancer Outcomes**
Winawer et al,[43] 1993	1418	5.9	SIR 0.24 (95% CI, 0.08–0.56)
Zauber et al,[44] 2012	2602	15.8	SMR 0.47 (95% CI, 0.26–0.80)
Citarda et al,[45] 2001	1693	10.5	SIR 0.34 (95% CI, 0.23–0.63)
Jorgensen et al[46]	2041	1–24	Incidence RR 0.65 (95% CI, 0.43–0.95) Mortality RR 0.12 (95% CI, 0.03–0.36)
Schatzkin et al,[48] 2000	2079	3.1	Incidence 2.2 per 1000 person-years
Alberts et al,[47] 2000	1429	3	Incidence 2.4 per 1000 person-years
Robertson et al,[49] 2005	2915	1.74	Incidence 1.7 per 1000 person-years
Nishihara et al,[14] 2013	88,902	22	Incidence HR 0.57 (95% CI, 0.45–0.72) Mortality HR 0.32 (95% CI, 0.24–0.45)
Cottet et al,[55] 2012	5779	7.7	SIR 1.26 (95% CI, 1.01–1.56)
Loberg et al[56]	40,826	7.7	SMR 0.96 (95% CI, 0.87–1.06)
Coleman et al,[57] 2015	6972	0.5–10 y	SIR 2.85 (95% CI, 2.61–3.25)

incidence based on SEER data (standardized incidence ratio [SIR] for CRC, 0.98; 95% CI, 0.63–1.54).

There are many potential reasons for these discrepant findings.[50] First, the NPS included a small number of experienced endoscopists, and there was significant focus on ensuring complete adenoma clearance prior to enrollment: patients with adenomas larger than 3 cm were excluded, and approximately 13% of the cohort underwent more than 1 baseline colonoscopy. Second, there were important methodological differences, including duration of follow-up, distinction between prevalent and incident CRC cases, the characteristics and CRC risk of the groups chosen for comparison, and frequency of surveillance colonoscopies after the index procedure. Finally, the quality of colonoscopy, notably neoplasia detection and completeness of polypectomy, were likely a contributing factor. These studies were conducted in an era which preceded the recognition of the importance of colonoscopy quality and its impact on the risk of post-colonoscopy CRC (PCCRC).[51,52] Although information about endoscopists' adenoma detection rates and completeness of polypectomy are not available, the characteristics of the incident cancers reported in these studies strongly suggest that colonoscopy quality is a major factor, because most would qualify as interval or post-colonoscopy CRC based on current definitions. For example, in the NPS, 3 of 5 incident cancers were detected 3 years after the index procedure and all 9 cancers in the Wheat Bran Fiber Trial were found within 3 years, whereas 10 of 13 CRC in the Polyp Prevention Trial were judged to be due to missed cancer, incomplete polypectomy, or inadequate biopsy. In the combined chemoprevention trial, 17 of 19 CRC were detected within 4 years of the baseline colonoscopy and most were in the proximal colon.

The central importance of polypectomy quality is not a theoretic one. In the landmark Complete Adenoma Resection study,[53] investigators biopsied the margins of 346 polypectomy sites and found an incomplete resection rate of 10.1% (95% CI, 6.9%–13.3%), ranging from 6.5% to 22.7% among endoscopists. Larger polyps were more likely to be incompletely resected than smaller polyps (17.3% vs 6.8%). The incomplete resection rate of 10%, alarming enough by itself, is likely an underestimate of the true prevalence of this problem in clinical practice, because study endoscopists were aware that they were participating in research and that their performance was being scrutinized. It is currently estimated that between 10% and 25% of PCCRCs are due to incomplete polypectomy.

More recent studies have further highlighted the effect of polypectomy on CRC prevention and the importance of continued surveillance in select higher-risk patients. An administrative claims-based study from Ontario[54] assessed whether characteristics of endoscopists are associated with risk of PCCRC in 14,064 patients. In multivariate analyses, patients with proximal cancers undergoing colonoscopy by endoscopists who performed polypectomies at high rates had a lower risk of PCCRC. Compared with less than 10% polypectomy rate reference, the odds ratio (OR) was 0.52 if the polypectomy rate was 25% to 29% and 0.61 for rates greater than 30%. Conversely, distal CRC was not associated with polypectomy rate. A large prospective study[14] examined the association of colonoscopy and sigmoidoscopy with CRC incidence and mortality among 88,902 participants in the Nurses' Health Study and the Health Professionals Follow-up Study. In follow-up of over 22 years compared with patients who had not undergone lower endoscopy, the multivariate HRs for CRC among participants were 0.57 (95% CI, 0.45–0.72) after resection of adenomatous polyps, 0.60 (95% CI, 0.53–0.68) after negative sigmoidoscopy, and 0.44 (95% CI, 0.38–0.52) after negative colonoscopy. Polypectomy was associated with reduced distal CRC incidence (HR 0.40; 95% CI, 0.27–0.59), although proximal colon cancer incidence was not significantly different. One possible advantage of this study over the NPS is that the polypectomy and control groups were derived from the same background population, allowing more direct comparison of CRC incidence rates after polypectomy and adjustment for confounding factors.

A French population-based cohort study[55] investigated CRC incidence in 5779 patients with adenomas, followed for a median of 7.7 years. Compared with the general French population, 87 CRCs were diagnosed versus 69 expected, for a SIR of 1.26 (95% CI, 1.01–1.56). CRC risk depended on the features of the index adenoma and whether surveillance colonoscopy occurred: the SIR was 2.23 (95% CI, 1.67–2.92) for advanced adenomas compared with 0.68 (95% CI, 0.44–0.99) for nonadvanced adenomas. For advanced adenomas, the SIR decreased to 1.10 (95% CI, 0.62–1.82) for patients who underwent colonoscopic surveillance but increased to 4.26 (95% CI, 2.89–6.04) for those who did not.

A population-based study from Norway[56] followed a cohort of 40,826 patients who underwent resection of colorectal adenomas between 1993 and 2007 and who were followed for a median of 7.7 years. Compared with the general Norwegian population, 383 CRC deaths were recorded (398 expected) for a standardized mortality ratio (SMR) of 0.96 (95% CI,0.87–1.06). CRC mortality was increased in high-risk adenoma patients (SMR 1.16; 95% CI, 1.02–1.31), and decreased among those with low-risk adenomas (SMR 0.75; 95% CI, 0.63–0.88).

A study[57] based on a Northern Ireland polyp registry reported a nearly 3-fold increased CRC risk among 6972 adenoma patients, and the excess risk was associated with inadequate colon clearance and follow-up after polypectomy.

Additional insight can be gained from follow-up of the subgroup of nearly 16,000 participants who underwent colonoscopy after abnormal findings on sigmoidoscopy.[58] When stratified according to adenoma findings at colonoscopy, and after a median of 13 years of follow-up, CRC incidence rates (per 10,000 person-years) were 20.0 (95% CI, 15.3–24.7) for advanced adenoma, 9.1 (95% CI, 6.7–11.5) for nonadvanced adenoma, and 7.5 (95% CI, 5.8–9.7; n = 71) for no adenoma. Participants with advanced adenoma were approximately 2.5 times more likely to develop or die from CRC compared with participants with no adenoma. There were no significant differences in CRC incidence and mortality between participants with nonadvanced adenoma compared with no adenoma.

These analyses highlight 2 key points. First, there are seems to be an efficacy to effectiveness gap between polypectomy studies, which can be explained by patient selection, adequacy of baseline colorectal clearance, and endoscopist polypectomy skill and resection completeness. This gap can explain most of the discrepancies between the NPS gold standard and observational population-based studies, which are based on data from heterogeneous clinical practice settings. Second, stratification of patients after baseline polypectomy allows the identification of a higher-risk subgroup (with advanced lesions) for whom successful CRC prevention requires more intensive surveillance and a numerically larger subgroup with lower-risk polyps for whom CRC risk can be reduced to the level of, or lower than, expected background population rates.

REFERENCES

1. Fletcher R, Fletcher S, Wagner E. Clinical epidemiology the essentials. 3rd edition. Philadelphia: Lippincott Williams and Wilkins; 1996.

2. Gilbertsen VA, Knatterud GL, Lober PH, et al. Invasive carcinoma of the large intestine: a preventable disease? Surgery 1965;57:363–5.

3. Vogelstein B, Fearon ER, Hamilton SR, et al. Genetic alterations during colorectal-tumor development. N Engl J Med 1988;319:525–32.

4. Kahi CJ, Imperiale TF, Juliar BE, et al. Effect of screening colonoscopy on colorectal cancer incidence and mortality. Clin Gastroenterol Hepatol 2009;7:770–5 [quiz 711].

5. Lieberman DA, Weiss DG, Bond JH, et al. Use of colonoscopy to screen asymptomatic adults for colorectal cancer. Veterans Affairs Cooperative Study Group 380. N Engl J Med 2000;343:162–8.

6. Lieberman DA, Weiss DG, Harford WV, et al. Five-year colon surveillance after screening colonoscopy. Gastroenterology 2007;133:1077–85.

7. Doubeni CA, Corley DA, Quinn VP, et al. Effectiveness of screening colonoscopy in reducing the risk of death from right and left colon cancer: a large community-based study. Gut 2018;67(2):291–8.

8. Doubeni CA, Weinmann S, Adams K, et al. Screening colonoscopy and risk for incident late-stage colorectal cancer diagnosis in average-risk adults: a nested case-control study. Ann Intern Med 2013;158:312–20.

9. Brenner H, Chang-Claude J, Jansen L, et al. Reduced risk of colorectal cancer up to 10 years after screening, surveillance, or diagnostic colonoscopy. Gastroenterology 2014;146:709–17.

10. Brenner H, Chang-Claude J, Seiler CM, et al. Protection from colorectal cancer after colonoscopy: a population-based, case-control study. Ann Intern Med 2011;154:22–30.

11. Brenner H, Hoffmeister M, Arndt V, et al. Protection from right- and left-sided colorectal neoplasms after colonoscopy: population-based study. J Natl Cancer Inst 2010;102:89–95.

12. Baxter NN, Goldwasser MA, Paszat LF, et al. Association of colonoscopy and death from colorectal cancer. Ann Intern Med 2009;150:1–8.

13. Baxter NN, Warren JL, Barrett MJ, et al. Association between colonoscopy and colorectal cancer mortality in a US cohort according to site of cancer and colonoscopist specialty. J Clin Oncol 2012;30:2664–9.

14. Nishihara R, Wu K, Lochhead P, et al. Long-term colorectal-cancer incidence and mortality after lower endoscopy. N Engl J Med 2013;369:1095–105.

15. Lee JK, Jensen CD, Levin TR, et al. Long-term risk of colorectal cancer and related deaths after a colonoscopy with normal findings. JAMA Intern Med 2019;179(2):153–60.

16. Brenner H, Chang-Claude J, Seiler CM, et al. Long-term risk of colorectal cancer after negative colonoscopy. J Clin Oncol 2011;29:3761–7.

17. Lakoff J, Paszat LF, Saskin R, et al. Risk of developing proximal versus distal colorectal cancer after a negative colonoscopy: a population-based study. Clin Gastroenterol Hepatol 2008;6:1117–21 [quiz 1064].

18. Singh H, Turner D, Xue L, et al. Risk of developing colorectal cancer following a negative colonoscopy examination: evidence for a 10-year interval between colonoscopies. JAMA 2006;295:2366–73.

19. Samadder NJ, Pappas L, Boucherr KM, et al. Long-term colorectal cancer incidence after negative colonoscopy in the state of utah: the effect of family history. Am J Gastroenterol 2017;112:1439–47.

20. Dominitz JA, Robertson DJ, Ahnen DJ, et al. Colonoscopy vs. Fecal Immunochemical Test in Reducing Mortality From Colorectal Cancer (CONFIRM): rationale for study design. Am J Gastroenterol 2017;112:1736–46.

21. Kaminski MF, Bretthauer M, Zauber AG, et al. The NordICC Study: rationale and design of a randomized trial on colonoscopy screening for colorectal cancer. Endoscopy 2012;44:695–702.

22. Quintero E, Castells A, Bujanda L, et al. Colonoscopy versus fecal immunochemical testing in colorectal-cancer screening. N Engl J Med 2012;366:697–706.

23. Colonoscopy and FIT as colorectal cancer screening test in the average risk population [clinical trial]. Available at: www.clinicaltrials.gov/ct2/show/NCT02078804. Accessed January 18, 2019.

24. Siegel RL, Miller KD, Jemal A. Cancer statistics, 2016. CA Cancer J Clin 2016; 66:7–30.

25. Tsoi KKF, Hirai HW, Chan FCH, et al. Predicted increases in incidence of colorectal cancer in developed and developing regions, in association with ageing populations. Clin Gastroenterol Hepatol 2017;15:892–900.e4.

26. Welch HG, Robertson DJ. Colorectal cancer on the decline–why screening can't explain it all. N Engl J Med 2016;374:1605–7.

27. Siegel RL, Fedewa SA, Anderson WF, et al. Colorectal cancer incidence patterns in the United States, 1974-2013. J Natl Cancer Inst 2017;109(8). djw322.

28. Brenner H, Schrotz-King P, Holleczek B, et al. Declining bowel cancer incidence and mortality in Germany. Dtsch Arztebl Int 2016;113:101–6.

29. Hardcastle JD, Chamberlain JO, Robinson MH, et al. Randomised controlled trial of faecal-occult-blood screening for colorectal cancer. Lancet 1996;348:1472–7.

30. Jorgensen OD, Kronborg O, Fenger C. A randomised study of screening for colorectal cancer using faecal occult blood testing: results after 13 years and seven biennial screening rounds. Gut 2002;50:29–32.

31. Kronborg O, Fenger C, Olsen J, et al. Randomised study of screening for colorectal cancer with faecal-occult-blood test. Lancet 1996;348:1467–71.

32. Faivre J, Dancourt V, Lejeune C, et al. Reduction in colorectal cancer mortality by fecal occult blood screening in a French controlled study. Gastroenterology 2004; 126:1674–80.

33. Mandel JS, Bond JH, Church TR, et al. Reducing mortality from colorectal cancer by screening for fecal occult blood. Minnesota Colon Cancer Control Study. N Engl J Med 1993;328:1365–71.

34. Shaukat A, Mongin SJ, Geisser MS, et al. Long-term mortality after screening for colorectal cancer. N Engl J Med 2013;369:1106–14.

35. Mandel JS, Church TR, Bond JH, et al. The effect of fecal occult-blood screening on the incidence of colorectal cancer. N Engl J Med 2000;343:1603–7.

36. Scholefield JH, Moss SM, Mangham CM, et al. Nottingham trial of faecal occult blood testing for colorectal cancer: a 20-year follow-up. Gut 2012;61:1036–40.

37. Elmunzer BJ, Hayward RA, Schoenfeld PS, et al. Effect of flexible sigmoidoscopy-based screening on incidence and mortality of colorectal cancer: a systematic review and meta-analysis of randomized controlled trials. PLoS Med 2012;9: e1001352.

38. Holme O, Bretthauer M, Fretheim A, et al. Flexible sigmoidoscopy versus faecal occult blood testing for colorectal cancer screening in asymptomatic individuals. Cochrane Database Syst Rev 2013;(9):CD009259.

39. Atkin WS, Edwards R, Kralj-Hans I, et al. Once-only flexible sigmoidoscopy screening in prevention of colorectal cancer: a multicentre randomised controlled trial. Lancet 2010;375:1624–33.

40. Atkin W, Wooldrage K, Parkin DM, et al. Long term effects of once-only flexible sigmoidoscopy screening after 17 years of follow-up: the UK Flexible Sigmoidoscopy Screening randomised controlled trial. Lancet 2017;389:1299–311.

41. Schoen RE, Pinsky PF, Weissfeld JL, et al. Colorectal-cancer incidence and mortality with screening flexible sigmoidoscopy. N Engl J Med 2012;366:2345–57.
42. Brenner H, Stock C, Hoffmeister M. Effect of screening sigmoidoscopy and screening colonoscopy on colorectal cancer incidence and mortality: systematic review and meta-analysis of randomised controlled trials and observational studies. BMJ 2014;348:g2467.
43. Winawer SJ, Zauber AG, Ho MN, et al. Prevention of colorectal cancer by colonoscopic polypectomy. The National Polyp Study Workgroup. N Engl J Med 1993; 329:1977–81.
44. Zauber AG, Winawer SJ, O'Brien MJ, et al. Colonoscopic polypectomy and long-term prevention of colorectal-cancer deaths. N Engl J Med 2012;366:687–96.
45. Citarda F, Tomaselli G, Capocaccia R, et al. Efficacy in standard clinical practice of colonoscopic polypectomy in reducing colorectal cancer incidence. Gut 2001; 48:812–5.
46. Jorgensen OD, Kronborg O, Fenger C, et al. Influence of long-term colonoscopic surveillance on incidence of colorectal cancer and death from the disease in patients with precursors (adenomas). Acta Oncol 2007;46:355–60.
47. Alberts DS, Martinez ME, Roe DJ, et al. Lack of effect of a high-fiber cereal supplement on the recurrence of colorectal adenomas. Phoenix Colon Cancer Prevention Physicians' Network. N Engl J Med 2000;342:1156–62.
48. Schatzkin A, Lanza E, Corle D, et al. Lack of effect of a low-fat, high-fiber diet on the recurrence of colorectal adenomas. Polyp Prevention Trial Study Group. N Engl J Med 2000;342:1149–55.
49. Robertson DJ, Greenberg ER, Beach M, et al. Colorectal cancer in patients under close colonoscopic surveillance. Gastroenterology 2005;129:34–41.
50. Hewett DG, Kahi CJ, Rex DK. Does colonoscopy work? J Natl Compr Canc Netw 2010;8:67–76 [quiz 77].
51. Corley DA, Jensen CD, Marks AR, et al. Adenoma detection rate and risk of colorectal cancer and death. N Engl J Med 2014;370:1298–306.
52. Kaminski MF, Regula J, Kraszewska E, et al. Quality indicators for colonoscopy and the risk of interval cancer. N Engl J Med 2010;362:1795–803.
53. Pohl H, Srivastava A, Bensen SP, et al. Incomplete polyp resection during colonoscopy-results of the complete adenoma resection (CARE) study. Gastroenterology 2013;144:74–80.e1.
54. Baxter NN, Sutradhar R, Forbes SS, et al. Analysis of administrative data finds endoscopist quality measures associated with postcolonoscopy colorectal cancer. Gastroenterology 2011;140:65–72.
55. Cottet V, Jooste V, Fournel I, et al. Long-term risk of colorectal cancer after adenoma removal: a population-based cohort study. Gut 2012;61:1180–6.
56. Løberg M, Kalager M, Holme Ø. Long-term colorectal-cancer mortality after adenoma removal. N Engl J Med 2014;371:799–807.
57. Coleman HG, Loughrey MB, Murray LJ, et al. Colorectal cancer risk following adenoma removal: a large prospective population-based cohort study. Cancer Epidemiol Biomarkers Prev 2015;24:1373–80.
58. Click B, Pinsky PF, Hickey T, et al. Association of colonoscopy adenoma findings with long-term colorectal cancer incidence. JAMA 2018;319:2021–31.

Assessing the Quality of Polypectomy and Teaching Polypectomy

Anna M. Duloy, MD[a], Rajesh N. Keswani, MD, MS[b],*

KEYWORDS

- Polypectomy • Competence • Quality • Teaching

KEY POINTS

- Despite known variability, polypectomy competence is rarely reported and quality metrics for this skill are lacking.
- Methods to assess polypectomy competence include assessment tools, such as the direct observation of polypectomy skills, and measurement of polypectomy outcomes, such as complete resection rates.
- Learning curves in polypectomy and the optimal approach to teaching polypectomy have not yet been established.

 Video content accompanies this article at http://www.giendo.theclinics.com.

INTRODUCTION

Colonoscopy with polypectomy is associated with a reduced risk of developing colorectal cancer.[1,2] Accordingly, there has been a significant emphasis on improving the detection of colorectal polyps through training and feedback.[1,3–5] In contrast, there is comparatively little work focused on assessing competence in colon polyp resection and training in optimal polypectomy techniques. Importantly, ineffective polypectomy technique may lead to incomplete polyp resection, increased complication rates, interval colorectal cancer, and costly referral to surgery.[6–8] Although polypectomy is essential to colorectal cancer prevention, competence is rarely reported and quality metrics for this skill are lacking. The few existing data suggest that polypectomy

Disclosure Statement: A.M. Duloy has nothing to disclose. R.N. Keswani has the following disclosures: Boston Scientific, Consultant; Medtronic, Consultant; and Motus-GI, Consultant.
[a] Division of Gastroenterology and Hepatology, University of Colorado Anschutz Medical Center, 1635, Aurora CT, Aurora, CO 80045, USA; [b] Department of Gastroenterology and Hepatology, Northwestern University, 676 North Street Clair, Suite 1400, Chicago, IL 60611, USA
* Corresponding author.
E-mail address: rajman@gmail.com

Gastrointest Endoscopy Clin N Am 29 (2019) 587–601
https://doi.org/10.1016/j.giec.2019.06.001
1052-5157/19/© 2019 Elsevier Inc. All rights reserved.

competence varies widely between colonoscopists, and interventions to improve polypectomy quality are needed.[6,9]

To ensure high-quality polypectomy technique is taught and practiced, what constitutes a competent polypectomy first must be defined. An overview of optimal polypectomy techniques is reviewed elsewhere in this issue. Once the components of high-quality polypectomy have been established, feasible methods must be determined to assess polypectomy competence (specifically, which assessment tools can be used), the current quality of polypectomy in trainees and practicing gastroenterologists, and effective methods to teach/remediate polypectomy skills.

ASSESSING THE QUALITY OF POLYPECTOMY

In the United States, formal assessments of polypectomy competence have not traditionally been a part of gastroenterology training programs. Similarly, there are no specific professional society guidelines suggesting evaluation of polypectomy performance among practicing physicians. In the American Society for Gastrointestinal Endoscopy (ASGE) privileging and credentialing guidelines,[10] a practitioner is expected to be able to competently perform snare polypectomy; however, how polypectomy competence should be defined remains unclear. Based on the usual tenets of high-quality medical care, a competent polypectomy would be expected to be safe (minimizing adverse events), efficient (occurring in a reasonable amount of time), and effective (removing all neoplastic tissue), while ideally minimizing costs.

The goals of polypectomy assessment tools are to objectively measure 1 or more of these core high-quality polypectomy concepts (eg, effective or safe polypectomy) in a feasible manner. Although a few tools have been developed, studies assessing polypectomy competence using these tools are limited. The existing tools are summarized, with an overview of the concepts and data supporting their use.

Polypectomy Competence Assessment Tools

Direct observation of polypectomy skills tool

The direct observation of polypectomy skills (DOPyS) tool was developed in response to a paucity of tools to measure polypectomy competence and has since been validated.[11–13] DOPyS is designed for the assessment of both live and videotaped polypectomy and includes 34 individual components and a global assessment scale (overall polypectomy competence) **(Fig. 1)**. A few of the components are only applicable to a live assessment of polypectomy. The remaining parameters are broken down into (1) preprocedural or general skills that are applicable to all polyps, (2) specific skills required depending on the morphology of the polyp (pedunculated vs sessile), and (3) postpolypectomy skills applicable to all polyps. Each of the individual parameters and the global scale are scored from 1 to 4, with scores of 1 (accepted standards not yet met with frequent uncorrected errors) or 2 (some standards not yet met, aspects to be improved, and some errors uncorrected) indicating a lack of competence and scores of 3 (competent and safe, no uncorrected errors) or 4 (highly skilled performance) denoting competence. The tool's validity and feasibility were established using video recordings of polypectomies performed by experienced endoscopists and have been shown to reliably differentiate polypectomies performed by endoscopists of varying levels of experience. The skills assessed focus on effective and safe removal of polyps; however, to the authors' knowledge, there currently are no data to correlate DOPyS scores with specific polypectomy outcomes, such as incomplete polyp resection or postpolypectomy adverse events.

DOPyS: Polypectomy Assessment Score Sheet

Date:_____

Assessor:_____

Endoscopist:_____

Case ID:_____

A separate sheet should be used for each case. Up to five polyps from one patient may be documents on the same DOPyS score sheet.

Scale and Criteria Key

4	Highly skilled performance
3	Competent and safe throughout procedure, no uncorrected errors
2	Some standards not yet met, aspects to be improved, some errors uncorrected
1	Accepted standards not yet met, frequent errors uncorrected
N/A	Not applicable/Not assessable

Generic	Polyp 1	Polyp 2	Polyp 3	Polyp 4	Polyp 5
Optimising view of / access to the polyp:					
1. Attempts to achieve optimal polyp position					
2. Optimises view by aspiration/insufflation/wash					
3. Determines full extent of lesion (+/- use of adjunctive techniques eg, bubble breaker, NBI, dye spray etc) if appropriate					
4. Uses appropriate polypectomy technique (eg, taking into account site in colon)					
5. Adjusts/stabilises scope position					
6. Checks all polypectomy equipment (forceps,snare,clips loops) available					
7. Checks (or asks assistant to) snare closure prior to introduction into the scope					
8. Clear instructions to and utilisation of endoscopy staff					
9. Checks diathermy settings are appropriate					
10. Photo-documents pre and post polypectomy					
Stalked polyps: Generic, then					
11. Applies prophylactic haemostatic measures if deemed appropriate					
12. Selects appropriate snare size					
13. Directs snare accurately over polyp head					
14. Correctly selects en-bloc or piecemeal removal depending on size					
15. Advances snare sheath towards stalk as snare closed					
16. Places snare at appropriate position on the stalk					
17. Mobilises polyp to ensure appropriate amount of tissue is trapped within snare					
18. Applies appropriate degree of diathermy					
Sessile lesions / Endoscopic mucosal resection: Generic, then					
19. Adequate sub mucosal injection using appropriate injection technique, maintaining views					
20. Only proceeds if the lesion lifts adequately					
21. Selects appropriate snare size					
22. Directs snare accurately over the lesion					
23. Correctly selects en-bloc or piecemeal removal depending on size					
24. Appropriate positioning of snare over lesion as snare closed					
25. Ensures appropriate amount of tissue is trapped within snare					
26. Tents lesion gently away from the mucosa					
27. Uses cold snare technique or applies appropriate diathermy, as applicable					
28. Ensures adequate haemostasis prior to further resection					
Post polypectomy					
29. Examines remnant stalk/polyp base					
30. Identifies and appropriately treats residual polyp					
31. Identifies bleeding and performs adequate endoscopic haemostasis if appropriate					
32. Retrieves, or attempts retrieval of polyp					
33. Checks for retrieval of polyp					
34. Places tattoo competently, where appropriate					
Polyp size	mm	mm	mm	mm	mm
Polyp site: C/AC/TC/DC/SC/Rectum					
Overall Competency at Polypectomy: 4/3/2/1					
Comments:					

Fig. 1. DOPyS tool.

Cold snare polypectomy assessment tool

A majority of polyps encountered in practice are diminutive, and these polyps are most effectively removed using a cold snare. In response to this, a tool was recently developed and validated to specifically assess competence in cold snare polypectomy.[14] The cold snare polypectomy assessment tool (CSPAT) was derived from the DOPyS but includes several new metrics unique to cold snare polypectomy. In total, the tool includes 12 metrics plus a global competence score designed for video-based assessments of cold snare polypectomy (**Table 1**). Like the DOPyS, each of the individual parameters and the global scale are scored from 1 to 4. Scores of 1 (standards not met) or 2 (some standards not met, uncorrected errors) indicate a lack of competence and scores of 3 (competent and safe, no uncorrected errors) or 4 (highly skilled)

Table 1
Cold snare polypectomy assessment tool

	Highly Skilled (Perfect) 4	Competent and Safe, No Uncorrected Errors (Adequate) 3	Some Standards Not Yet Met, Aspects to be Improved, Some Errors Uncorrected (Suboptimal) 2	Accepted Standards Not Met, Frequent Errors Uncorrected (Unacceptable) 1	Not Applicable/ Assessable N/A
1. Achieves optimal polyp position	Ensures good polyp position (5:00–6:00 position) with no errors during entire polypectomy	Maintains polyp at 5:00–6:00 position during most of polypectomy with attempts at position correction	Does not maintain polyp at 5:00–6:00 position. Few attempts made at position correction	Does not maintain polyp in the optimal position at any time during the procedure	
2. Optimizes view by aspiration/insufflation/ wash	Maintains clear polyp views throughout the procedure	Attempts to obtain clear polyp views through aspiration, insufflation, and lens wash	Clear polyp views not maintained	Poor polyp views throughout the procedure with no attempts at correction	
3. Adjusts/stabilizes scope position	Maintains stable colonoscope position throughout polypectomy	Adjusts and stabilizes colonoscope position before polypectomy	Colonoscope not stabilized adequately. Little or no attempts made to reposition scope	Unstable colonoscope position throughout procedure with no attempts made at correction	
4. Directs snare accurately over the lesion	Steers snare accurately over the lesion head with no errors	Steers snare accurately over the lesion head with minimal difficulty	Clumsy steering of snare over the lesion head	Clumsy steering of snare causing mucosal injury	
5. Anchors sheath of snare several mm distal (downstream) to polyp	Efficiently and accurately positions and anchors snare several millimeters distal to polyp	Achieves adequate positioning of snare several mm distal to polyp, though with some inefficiency	Does not anchor sheath distal to polyp. Polypectomy may be adequate but without border of normal tissue	Does not anchor sheath distal to polyp resulting in residual polyp tissue	
6. Keeps tools close to scope	Keeps tool close to scope at all times	Keeps tool close to scope most of the time and in a way that does not preclude adequate polypectomy	Does not keep tool close to scope, but achieves adequate polypectomy	Does not keep tool close to scope, resulting in inadequate polypectomy	

7. Appropriate positioning of snare over lesion as snare closed	Accurately positions snare over lesion as snare closed gradually	Advances snare sheath in a controlled fashion toward stalk as snare is closed	Closes snare too rapidly or in an uncontrolled fashion	Closes snare too rapidly, cutting/shearing through the polyp tissue
8. Ensures appropriate amount of tissue is trapped within snare	Always ensures no additional tissue is trapped within snare	Ensures no additional tissue is trapped within snare	Does not ensure that additional tissue is not trapped within snare.	Does not check for additional tissue trapped within snare before resecting polyp
9. Ensures rim of normal tissue is resected around polyp	Rim of normal tissue around entire polyp	Rim of normal tissue around most of polyp, but some areas resected at polyp border, adequate polypectomy	Most of polyp border without normal rim of tissue	No normal tissue around polyp resulting in residual polyp
10. Examines postpolypectomy site	Full visualization of postpolypectomy site using water jet to clear debris/blood	Visualization of postpolypectomy site but some residual debris/blood	Suboptimal visualization of postpolypectomy site where observer cannot tell whether resection was complete	No visualization of postpolypectomy site
11. Identifies and appropriately treats residual polyp	Identifies and resects any residual tissue accurately	Identifies and resects any residual tissue	Does not adequately identify or treat visible residual polyp tissue	Leaves residual polyp tissue behind
12. Retrieves, or attempts, retrieval of polyp	Retrieves polyp by using method appropriate to polyp/size	Retrieves or attempts retrieval of polyp. May not use method appropriate to polyp/size	Inadequate attempt at retrieval of polyp	No attempts made at polyp retrieval

Rate the overall polypectomy _____

Polypectomy time: _____

Polyp size: _____

Polyp morphology: ☐ Sessile ☐ Flat ☐ Pedunculated

indicate competence. Scoring criteria for each assessment anchor also are included in the tool. Experts in cold snare polypectomy used the CSPAT tool to evaluate preselected videos that were previously evaluated using the DOPyS tool. The tool showed a moderate degree of correlation to DOPyS scores assigned to the same videos, suggesting external validity.

The CSPAT is a more abbreviated assessment tool, making it less cumbersome and time consuming to use and includes novel skills specific to cold snare polypectomy. The CSPAT largely assumes, however, that the correct technique is chosen to remove the polyp and, therefore, unlike the DOPyS, does not address and allow for feedback on whether the correct polypectomy technique was chosen. Furthermore, the CSPAT is not intended for use to assess the quality of resection of colon polyps removed after submucosal lift and/or with the use of cautery.

Assessment of competency in endoscopy tool for colonoscopy

The assessment of competence in endoscopy (ACE) tool was developed by the ASGE to evaluate the cognitive and technical aspects of colonoscopy.[15] Two of the 13 questions address trainee performance on therapeutic interventions, including polypectomy. If polypectomy was performed, trainees are evaluated from 1 to 4 on 2 questions: What was the fellow's participation in the therapeutic maneuver (1—novice, performed with significant hands-on assistance or coaching; 2—intermediate, performed with minor hands-on assistance or significant coaching; 3—advanced, performed independently, with minor coaching; or 4—superior, performed independently without coaching)? and What was the fellow's knowledge of the therapeutic tool (1—novice, unsure of the possible tool indicated or settings for pathology encountered; 2—intermediate, able to identify possible appropriate tool choices but not sure which would be ideal; 3—advanced, independently selects the correct tool yet needs coaching on settings; or 4—superior, independently identifies correct tool and settings as applicable)? The questions likely approximate a global assessment of polypectomy skill. If a trainee is found deficient in polypectomy competence, however, the tool does not provide specific actionable areas for remediation (in contrast to the DOPyS and CSPAT, which highlight performance on multiple specific polypectomy skills).

Polypectomy Outcomes

Measuring polypectomy outcomes, such as postpolypectomy adverse event rates and rates of incomplete polypectomy, are another way to assess polypectomy competence among practicing gastroenterologists, although potentially more costly and resource intensive than the previously discussed competence assessment tools. The ASGE recommends evaluation of postprocedure quality indicators among practicing gastroenterologists, including the incidence of perforation and postpolypectomy bleeding.[16] Perforation rates greater than 1 in 500 overall or greater than 1 in 1000 in screening patients and postpolypectomy bleeding rates greater than 1% should prompt an assessment of endoscopist polypectomy technique. Given the infrequent nature of these adverse events, however, it is unlikely that a statistically significant variation in adverse event rates would be identified between colonoscopists.

Biopsies of the postpolypectomy site allow for the ultimate evaluation of polypectomy competence, although this technique requires additional procedural time, labor, and costs and may not be feasible in most practice settings. Incomplete polypectomy rates among practicing gastroenterologists range from 6.5% to 22.6%, even for small polyps.[6] In a prospective study of 1427 patients, approximately 10% of polyps were found to be incompletely resected, as evidenced by residual polyp on biopsy of the polypectomy site after completion of polypectomy.[6] This rate was even greater

(31%) for serrated polyps. The rate of incomplete resection increased with polyp size and was highly variable among endoscopists, ranging from 7% to 23%. Studies that assess for a correlation between incomplete polypectomy resection rates and competence scores (using tools like the DOPyS and CSPAT) will be critically important.

Polypectomy Competence Among Trainees

Studies evaluating trainee competence at polypectomy are limited. In a small prospective study, 8 trainees from the Netherlands were video-recorded while performing 5 consecutive polypectomies.[17] All of the fellows had performed at least 100 colonoscopies and at least 20 polypectomies. Of the 40 evaluated polyps, 25 measured 1 mm to 5 mm, 9 measured 6 mm to 9 mm, and 6 polyps were 15 mm. More than half of the polyps were removed with a lift plus hot snare polypectomy (23/40, 58%), whereas the remainder were removed with cold snare (28%) or a lift plus cold snare (15%). The polypectomies were graded using the DOPyS, and 78% (31/40) received a failing or not competent DOPyS score (DOPyS score of 1 or 2). In a study evaluating 131 trainees in the United Kingdom,[18] 94% of trainees achieved level 1 polypectomy competence (defined as overall scores of 3 or 4 in their last 4 consecutive DOPyS for polyps <1 cm) within 3 years of their first DOPyS assessment, but only 50% achieved level 2 competence (defined as overall scores of 3 or 4 in their last 4 consecutive DOPyS for polyps [1–2 cm]) in the same time period.

Two studies have looked at the number of polypectomies required for trainees to achieve competence. One of these studies found that trainees achieve competence in colonoscopic polypectomy (defined as an en bloc resection and polypectomy time within twice the median polypectomy time of 3 experienced colonoscopists) after 250 polypectomies.[19] The second study found that the complete resection rate of fellows was comparable to that of experts after 300 hot snare polypectomies.[20]

Polypectomy Competence Among Independent Colonoscopists

There also are few data on polypectomy competence among practicing colonoscopists. The DOPyS tool was used to assess colon polypectomy competence among 13 high-volume screening colonoscopists at an academic medical center in the United States.[9] Only 64% of all polypectomies were rated as competent. Polypectomy was performed more competently for polyps less than 6 mm (70%) than polyps greater than or equal to 6 mm (50%; $P = .03$). Moreover, there was significant variability in polypectomy competence among the gastroenterologists, with overall polypectomy competence rates (as measured by the DOPyS), ranging from 30% to 90%.

The correlation between polypectomy competence and established colonoscopy quality metrics (adenoma detection rate [ADR] and withdrawal time [WT]) also was evaluated to determine whether high-performing detectors (ie, higher ADRs) were high-performing resectors (ie, higher DOPyS scores). Importantly, polypectomy competence rates did not significantly correlate with historical ADRs ($r = 0.4$; $P = .2$) or historical WTs ($r = 0.2$; $P = .5$). These findings suggest that even if gastroenterologists are skillful at detecting polyps, they are not necessarily competent at removing them. Additionally, colonoscopists with a quick WT may still be skillful at polyp removal. Key performance metrics of colonoscopy quality, therefore, cannot be used as surrogate markers for competence in polypectomy.

Specific skills that colonoscopists were deficient in were further assessed. Optimal polypectomy position and a stable endoscope position were competently achieved in 61% and 58% of polypectomies, respectively, and the colonoscopists sufficiently evaluated the polypectomy site for remnant tissue in only 57% of polypectomies. Among sessile lesions removed by snare, colonoscopists chose the correct snare size and competently positioned the snare over the polyp in 73% of polyps, but an appropriate amount of tissue was competently resected in only 50% of polyps. Additionally, there were low rates of submucosal lift polypectomy in the removal of polyps greater than or equal to 6 mm. A submucosal lift was used in 2 of 19 (11%) of Paris IIa and IIb polyps greater than or equal to 6 mm and in 0 Paris Is polyps greater than or equal to 6 mm. Consequently, several of these polyps (all ≤15 mm) were removed piecemeal and/or residual polyp was visualized after polypectomy completion.

TEACHING AND REMEDIATING POLYPECTOMY
Society Guidelines and Scientific Literature

It is important for trainees and practicing colonoscopists to understand the scientific underpinning of high-quality polypectomy. Society guidelines and published literature provide useful and evidence-based frameworks to guide best practices for polypectomy. The European Society of Gastrointestinal Endoscopy has published guidelines that provide detailed recommendations on which polypectomy techniques should be used based on polyp size and morphology, with the relevant supporting literature.[21,22] Similarly, the ASGE has published a technical review on the endoscopic management of colon polyps.[23] For diminutive polyps (1–5 mm), cold snare polypectomy is suggested; for small polyps (6–9 mm), recommended approaches include cold or hot snare polypectomy; and for larger polyps, suggested techniques vary based on the type of polyp. Unfortunately, it is clear that many physicians remain unaware of best practices. In prior studies, use of low-quality practices (eg, piecemeal cold forceps polypectomy or hot biopsy forceps polypectomy) remain common.[9,24–26] Thus, an important component to teaching high-quality polypectomy is developing novel ways to disseminate best practice. Existing methods to disseminate best practices include textbooks, original research studies, review articles, society-generated electronic mail with video tips, social media, and online video libraries.

Current State of Polypectomy Training

There has been a concerted effort to transition endoscopic training from volume-based apprenticeship to competency based medical education.[27] Multiple endoscopic curricula[28,29] and competency assessment tools[13,15,30] have been developed to assist fellowship programs in standardizing endoscopic curricula and evaluating competence in endoscopy; however, training in polypectomy during gastroenterology fellowship is not standardized in the United States, with some trainees receiving little formal guidance before being expected to perform polypectomy indepdendently.[27,31] Although the Accreditation Council for Graduate Medical Education provides a framework,[32] the cognitive and hands-on teaching of endoscopic procedures, in particular polypectomy, varies broadly and most training programs lack systematic training in polypectomy.

There is significant variability in polypectomy training worldwide and the optimal (most effective) training approach has not been well defined. It is unclear what proportions of polypectomy training should consist of didactics, use of simulation/ex vivo models, watching experts, and supervised hands-on polypectomy. There are few data on the efficacy of each of these interventions, leading to varying practices across institutions and countries. In an international survey of 262 trainees and 348 trainers,[33] most trainees reported a lack of training for resection of large polyps and minimal to no training in endoscopic mucosal resection. Just over half (53%) of trainees report being formally assessed on their polypectomy technique, with 49% reporting that the polypectomy assessment process was not documented in any form. Additionally, a minority of trainers had received formal training on how to teach fellows and trainers from most countries reported a lack of specific national guidelines on polypectomy training and assessment, with only 51% using a formal framework when assessing trainee polypectomy performance. In another study, only 60% of trainees had ever been assessed in polypectomy.[34] These studies highlight the alarming variability in how trainees are taught and assessed in polypectomy.

Studies assessing which training methods most effectively improve trainee polypectomy competence are limited. In a study of 8 gastroenterology fellows, a lecture-based training course (3 lectures were given by polypectomy experts on polyp characterization, including morphology, pit pattern, endoscopic assessment of histology, and on-site decision making regarding therapy; polypectomy technique with video examples of correct and incorrect technique; and the management and recognition of polypectomy complications) did not result in an improvement in overall competence scores as assessed by the DOPyS.[17] Whether alternative lecture-based approaches would be effective is unknown. The Improving Competency and Metrics for Polypectomy Skills Using Evaluation Tools and Video Feedback (COMPLETE) study is an ongoing multicenter randomized study that is evaluating learning curves in cold snare polypectomy among trainees.[35] Using the DOPyS, the study is evaluating trainee competence in cold snare polypectomy and determining the role of video-based feedback and teaching modules on incomplete resection rates and competence among trainees. It is currently unknown, however, whether this laborious intervention can effectively improve polypectomy competence. These data highlight the need for a standardized, evidence-based approach to teaching and assessing polypectomy among gastroenterology trainees.

In contrast to most countries where polypectomy training is heterogenous between institutions, formalized polypectomy assessment is now a mandatory part of training and the colonoscopy certification process for endoscopists planning to perform bowel cancer screening procedures in the United Kingdom. To obtain provisional certification, trainees must demonstrate competence ($\geq$3 on DOPyS scoring) in the removal of polyps less than 1 cm. Trainees can apply for full accreditation when their DOPyS scores are greater than or equal to 3 on more than 90% of their last 4 DOPyS assessments for polyps greater than 1 cm. The introduction of this requirement resulted in a significant increase in the number of logged polypectomy assessments ($P<.001$) and experience in endoscopic mucosal resection ($P<.001$) among trainees.[36] There is an urgent need for similar standardization in teaching programs in the United States and across the world.

Assessment and Remediation of Polypectomy Quality in Practicing Colonoscopists

The key limitation to assessing polypectomy competence in independent practitioners is identifying a feasible tool to use. As discussed previously, there are 2 potential methods to assess polypectomy competence—use of a validated assessment tool (eg, DOPyS or CSPAT) or biopsy of the polypectomy site to evaluate for residual neoplasia. It is unclear, however, whether these methods can be broadly utilized outside of a research setting or focused quality improvement efforts, given the time and/or costs associated with their use. Once inadequate polypectomy technique is established in an independent colonoscopist, however, there are several available options for remediation.

Report cards

A single study has evaluated the effect of a report card with teaching videos on polypectomy competence among attending gastroenterologist.[37] Eleven colonoscopists at an academic institution were given individualized report cards plus instructional videos after a baseline assessment of polypectomy quality. Ten polypectomies per colonoscopist were graded using the DOPyS and the detailed scores were given to them on a report card (**Fig. 2**), along with 9 instructional videos with narration, each 2 minutes to 5 minutes in length, that demonstrated optimal and poor technique for the following skills: uses appropriate polypectomy technique; attempts to achieve optimal polyp position; determines full extent of lesion; adjusts/stabilizes scope position; examines remnant stalk/polyp base; identifies and appropriately treats residual polyp; submucosal injection and lift; selecting appropriate snare size and appropriate positioning of snare as it is closed; and ensuring adequate tissue is removed (Videos 1 and 2). The colonoscopists were video-recorded before the report cards were distributed (pre-report card) and after their distribution (post-report card). The mean DOPyS score significantly increased between the pre-report card and post-report card phases (2.7 ± 0.9 vs 3.0 ± 0.8; $P = .01$). This improvement was observed for diminutive polyps (2.7 ± 0.9 vs 3.3 ± 0.8; $P<.001$) but not for larger ($\geq$6 mm) polyps (2.7 ± 0.7 vs 2.4 ± 0.9; $P = .3$). The rate of competent polypectomy significantly improved from the pre-report card to post-report card phases (56% vs 69%; $P = .04$). Again, this improvement was seen for diminutive polyps (57% vs 81%; $P = .001$) but not for larger polyps (55% vs 36%; $P = .02$). Most polyps were removed by cold snare in both phases; however, cold snare use increased significantly between the pre-report card and post-report card phases (58% vs 76%; $P = .001$). Additionally, the rate of piecemeal polypectomy significantly decreased (40% vs 21%; $P = .001$). These results suggest that a polypectomy report card and video-based teaching can improve competence among attending gastroenterologists. Different education strategies may be necessary, however, for improving the resection of larger polyps. Furthermore, this is a time-consuming intervention that may not be widely feasible.

Simulation
Simulators can provide an effective skills training platform without the risk of complications for patients. It is unclear, however, whether such training translates into improved outcomes in clinical endoscopic practice and, in most cases, simulators are expensive, require specialized facilities, and allow for training in a limited number of techniques. Studies supporting the use of simulators for polypectomy are limited. The Welsh Institute for Minimal Access Therapy colonoscopy suitcase is an ex vivo porcine simulator for polypectomy that has shown content validity for training in polypectomy skills.[38,39] The model does not have inbuilt parameters for assessment, and retrospective assessments of video-recorded performances using tools, such as the DOPyS, must be used. The model was validated for snare polypectomy and showed that DOPyS scores obtained on the simulator correlate with the real-life level of expertise of the user. Another simulator, the endoscopic part-task training box,[40] consists of 5 training modules, 1 of which is polypectomy. The operator must use a snare to circumferentially grasp polyps made of a malleable synthetic polymer located at fixed stations on the simulator's walls. With proper snare position, an electronic circuit is completed, and the user is awarded points. The training box differentiated between experience levels for the polypectomy task (novice, first-year fellow, second-year fellow, third-year fellow, and attending physician) and, for those participants who repeated the training box exercise, interval score improvement was seen over time. In another study, participants were randomized to receive 30-minute 1-on-1 hands-on skills training sessions on snare polypectomy and hot biopsy using an ex vivo model versus no hands on training.[41] Those participants receiving training on the polypectomy model had significantly higher skills assessment scores.

John Doe, MD

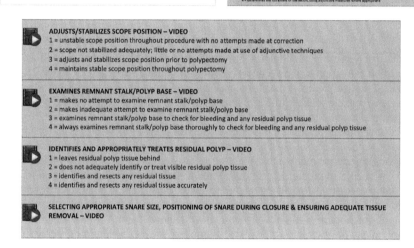

Direct Observation of Polypectomy Skills (DOPyS)
The DOPyS tool assesses several different polypectomy skills. Each skill is graded from 1–4, where a score of 1 = standards not met; 2 = some standards not met, uncorrected errors; 3 = competent and safe, no uncorrected errors and 4 = highly skilled. A score of 3 or greater denotes passing. Ten polypectomies per endoscopist were graded and a mean score and % pass was calculated for each polypectomy skill.

Your Scores
Your individual DOPyS scores are displayed in the following tables. Cohort scores are the mean scores of all 13 participating endoscopists.

Videos
Click on the links to view short educational videos that highlight examples of optimal technique (received high scores) and poor technique (received low scores) for DOPyS skills.

DOPyS SCORES	Your score	Your percent pass	Cohort score	Cohort percent pass	05th percentile score	50th percentile score	75th percentile score
Uses appropriate technique (1–4)	3.05	50%	3.22	70%	3.05	3.25	3.45
Attempts to achieve optimal polyp position (1–4)	3.25	80%	2.91	60.7%	2.80	2.85	3.20
Determines full extent of lesion (1–4)	2.90	80%	2.70	72.3%	2.60	2.80	2.90
Adjusts/stabilizes scope position (2–4)	3.00	70%	2.80	58.4%	2.65	2.80	3.00
Examines remnant stalk/polyp base (1–4)	2.60	40%	2.83	56.9%	2.60	2.85	2.95
Identifies and appropriately treats residual polyp (1–4)	2.50	40%	2.73	58.4%	2.50	2.75	3.10
Overall Performance (1–4)	2.75	60%	2.78	63.9%	2.55	2.75	3.00

USES APPROPRIATE TECHNIQUE – VIDEO
1 = inappropriate polypectomy technique; choice of technique is inappropriate or unsafe
2 = chooses inappropriate polypectomy technique
3 = uses appropriate polypectomy technique safely based on size, site, and morphology
4 = uses most appropriate polypectomy technique safely with no errors

ATTEMPTS TO ACHIEVE OPTIMAL POLYP POSITION – VIDEO
1 = does not maintain polyp in the optimal position at any time during the procedure
2 = does not maintain polyp at 5-6 o'clock position; few attempts made at position correction
3 = maintains polyp at 5-6 o'clock position with attempts at position correction
4 = ensures good polyp position (5-6 o'clock position) with no errors; attempts made at position correction throughout the procedure

DETERMINES FULL EXTENT OF LESION – VIDEO
1 = no attempts made at determining or visualising full extent of the polyp; attempts polypectomy on lesions which are unlikely to be endoscopically respectable
2 = does not determine or visualise full extent of the polyp or fails to recognize features suggestive of malignancy
3 = determines the full extent of the lesion, may not use adjunctive measures
4 = determines the full extent of the lesion, using adjunctive measures where appropriate

ADJUSTS/STABILIZES SCOPE POSITION – VIDEO
1 = unstable scope position throughout procedure with no attempts made at correction
2 = scope not stabilized adequately; little or no attempts made at use of adjunctive techniques
3 = adjusts and stabilizes scope position prior to polypectomy
4 = maintains stable scope position throughout polypectomy

EXAMINES REMNANT STALK/POLYP BASE – VIDEO
1 = makes no attempt to examine remnant stalk/polyp base
2 = makes inadequate attempt to examine remnant stalk/polyp base
3 = examines remnant stalk/polyp base to check for bleeding and any residual polyp tissue
4 = always examines remnant stalk/polyp base thoroughly to check for bleeding and any residual polyp tissue

IDENTIFIES AND APPROPRIATELY TREATS RESIDUAL POLYP – VIDEO
1 = leaves residual polyp tissue behind
2 = does not adequately identify or treat visible residual polyp tissue
3 = identifies and resects any residual tissue
4 = identifies and resects any residual tissue accurately

SELECTING APPROPRIATE SNARE SIZE, POSITIONING OF SNARE DURING CLOSURE & ENSURING ADEQUATE TISSUE REMOVAL – VIDEO

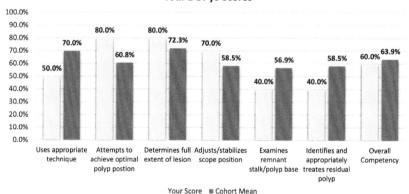

Your DOPyS Scores

Your Score ■ Cohort Mean

Fig. 2. Example polypectomy skills report card.

Videos

Videos are an increasingly utilized resource for on-demand learning of endoscopic procedures. There are a wide range of educational videos on polypectomy, which can be accessed online via YouTube, the ASGE video library, and VideoGIE. There are no data, however, showing that viewing of these videos has any demonstrable effect on polypectomy quality.

Hands-on courses

Courses offering hands-on training in polypectomy are available throughout the world and are hosted by industry, academic institutions, and professional gastroenterology societies. Many of these courses allow for supervised learning on animal models with expert trainers and teach attendees the most up-to-date and evidence-based techniques. Although these courses may demonstrate advanced techniques and offer tips and tricks to aid in self-improvement, there are not data, to the authors' knowledge, to suggest that these courses have an impact on polypectomy competence and/or can alter the actual polypectomy skills of attendees.

SUMMARY

Ineffective polypectomy technique may lead to incomplete polyp resection, high complication rates, interval colorectal cancer, and costly referral to surgery. Despite its central importance to endoscopy, training in polypectomy is not standardized nor has the most effective training approach been defined. Furthermore, despite known variability, polypectomy competence is rarely reported and quality metrics for this skill are lacking. Current methods to assess polypectomy competence include tools, such as the DOPyS, CSPAT, and the ACE tool for colonoscopy, and assessment of polypectomy outcomes, such as incomplete resection and bleeding rates. Use of these tools and/or measurement of outcomes among colonoscopists in independent practice and trainees is low, likely related to feasibility. There is a need for consensus on standardization of training and remediation in polypectomy; defining standards of competent polypectomy and how it is feasibly measured; and, the integration of polypectomy quality metrics into training programs and the accreditation process.

SUPPLEMENTARY DATA

Supplementary data related to this article can be found online at https://doi.org/10.1016/j.giec.2019.06.001.

REFERENCES

1. Corley DA, Jensen CD, Marks AR, et al. Adenoma detection rate and risk of colorectal cancer and death. N Engl J Med 2014;370(14):1298–306.

2. Zauber AG, Winawer SJ, O'Brien MJ, et al. Colonoscopic polypectomy and long-term prevention of colorectal-cancer deaths. N Engl J Med 2012;366(8):687–96.

3. Kaminski MF, Regula J, Kraszewska E, et al. Quality indicators for colonoscopy and the risk of interval cancer. N Engl J Med 2010;362(19):1795–803.

4. Kahi CJ, Ballard D, Shah AS, et al. Impact of a quarterly report card on colonoscopy quality measures. Gastrointest Endosc 2013;77(6):925–31.

5. Keswani RN, Yadlapati R, Gleason KM, et al. Physician report cards and implementing standards of practice are both significantly associated with improved screening colonoscopy quality. Am J Gastroenterol 2015;110(8):1134–9.

6. Pohl H, Srivastava A, Bensen SP, et al. Incomplete polyp resection during colonoscopy-results of the complete adenoma resection (CARE) study. Gastroenterology 2013;144(1):74–80.e1.

7. Aziz Aadam A, Wani S, Kahi C, et al. Physician assessment and management of complex colon polyps: a multicenter video-based survey study. Am J Gastroenterol 2014;109(9):1312–24.

8. Robertson DJ, Lieberman DA, Winawer SJ, et al. Colorectal cancers soon after colonoscopy: a pooled multicohort analysis. Gut 2014;63(6):949–56.

9. Duloy AM, Kaltenbach TR, Keswani RN. Assessing colon polypectomy competency and its association with established quality metrics. Gastrointest Endosc 2018;87(3):635–44.

10. ASGE Standards of Practice Committee, Faulx AL, Lightdale JR, et al. Guidelines for privileging, credentialing, and proctoring to perform GI endoscopy. Gastrointest Endosc 2017;85(2):273–81.

11. Gupta S, Anderson J, Bhandari P, et al. Development and validation of a novel method for assessing competency in polypectomy: direct observation of polypectomy skills. Gastrointest Endosc 2011;73(6):1232–9.e2.

12. Gupta S, Bassett P, Man R, et al. Validation of a novel method for assessing competency in polypectomy. Gastrointest Endosc 2012;75(3):568–75.

13. Barton JR, Corbett S, van der Vleuten CP, English Bowel Cancer Screening Programme, UK Joint Advisory Group for Gastrointestinal Endoscopy. The validity and reliability of a Direct Observation of Procedural Skills assessment tool: assessing colonoscopic skills of senior endoscopists. Gastrointest Endosc 2012; 75(3):591–7.

14. Patel S, Duloy A, Kaltenbach TR, et al. Mo1660 assessing competence in cold snare polypectomy: evaluation of a modified version of the direct observation of polypectomy skills (DOPYS) tool. Gastrointest Endosc 2018;87(6):AB466.

15. Committee AT, Sedlack RE, Coyle WJ, et al. ASGE's assessment of competency in endoscopy evaluation tools for colonoscopy and EGD. Gastrointest Endosc 2014;79(1):1–7.

16. Rex DK, Schoenfeld PS, Cohen J, et al. Quality indicators for colonoscopy. Gastrointest Endosc 2015;81(1):31–53.

17. van Doorn SC, Bastiaansen BA, Thomas-Gibson S, et al. Polypectomy skills of gastroenterology fellows: can we improve them? Endosc Int Open 2016;4(2): E182–9.

18. Rajendran A, Thomas-Gibson S, Bassett P, et al. PTU-006 Time to polypectomy competency in the uk: retrospective analysis of 1633 dopys from 131 trainees. Gut 2017;66(Suppl 2):A53.

19. Boo SJ, Jung JH, Park JH, et al. An adequate level of training for technically competent colonoscopic polypectomy. Scand J Gastroenterol 2015;50(7): 908–15.

20. Choi JM, Lee C, Park JH, et al. Complete resection of colorectal adenomas: what are the important factors in fellow training? Dig Dis Sci 2015;60(6):1579–88.

21. Kaminski MF, Thomas-Gibson S, Bugajski M, et al. Performance measures for lower gastrointestinal endoscopy: a European Society of Gastrointestinal Endoscopy (ESGE) quality improvement initiative. Endoscopy 2017;49(4):378–97.

22. Kaminski MF, Thomas-Gibson S, Bugajski M, et al. Performance measures for lower gastrointestinal endoscopy: a European Society of Gastrointestinal Endoscopy (ESGE) quality improvement initiative. United European Gastroenterol J 2017;5(3):309–34.

23. Burgess NG, Bahin FF, Bourke MJ. Colonic polypectomy (with videos). Gastrointest Endosc 2015;81(4):813–35.

24. Lee CK, Shim JJ, Jang JY. Cold snare polypectomy vs. Cold forceps polypectomy using double-biopsy technique for removal of diminutive colorectal polyps: a prospective randomized study. Am J Gastroenterol 2013;108(10):1593–600.

25. Efthymiou M, Taylor AC, Desmond PV, et al. Biopsy forceps is inadequate for the resection of diminutive polyps. Endoscopy 2011;43(4):312–6.

26. Hewett DG. Colonoscopic polypectomy: current techniques and controversies. Gastroenterol Clin North Am 2013;42(3):443–58.

27. Patel SG, Keswani R, Elta G, et al. Status of competency-based medical education in endoscopy training: a nationwide survey of US ACGME-accredited gastroenterology training programs. Am J Gastroenterol 2015;110(7):956–62.

28. Patel S, Rastogi A, Austin G, et al. Gastroenterology trainees can easily learn histologic characterization of diminutive colorectal polyps with narrow band imaging (NBI). Am J Gastroenterol 2012;107(Supplement 1):S807.

29. Higashi R, Uraoka T, Kato J, et al. Diagnostic accuracy of narrow-band imaging and pit pattern analysis significantly improved for less-experienced endoscopists after an expanded training program. Gastrointest Endosc 2010;72(1):127–35.

30. Vassiliou MC, Kaneva PA, Poulose BK, et al. Global assessment of gastrointestinal endoscopic skills (GAGES): a valid measurement tool for technical skills in flexible endoscopy. Surg Endosc 2010;24(8):1834–41.

31. Zanchetti DJ, Schueler SA, Jacobson BC, et al. Effective teaching of endoscopy: a qualitative study of the perceptions of gastroenterology fellows and attending gastroenterologists. Gastroenterol Rep (Oxf) 2016;4(2):125–30.

32. ACGME program requirements for graduate medical education in gastroenterology (internal medicine). Available at: https://www.acgme.org/Portals/0/PFAssets/ProgramRequirements/144_gastroenterology_2017-07-01.pdf. Accessed Decemeber 15, 2018.

33. Patel K, Rajendran A, Faiz O, et al. An international survey of polypectomy training and assessment. Endosc Int Open 2017;5(3):E190–7.

34. Haycock AV, Patel JH, Tekkis PP, et al. Evaluating changes in gastrointestinal endoscopy training over 5 years: closing the audit loop. Eur J Gastroenterol Hepatol 2010;22(3):368–73.

35. ClinicalTrials.gov. Improving competency and metrics for polypectomy skills using evaluation tools and video feedback (COMPLETE). Identifier: NCT03115008. Available at: https://clinicaltrials.gov/ct2/show/NCT03115008. Accessed December 15, 2018.

36. Patel K, Faiz O, Rutter M, et al. The impact of the introduction of formalised polypectomy assessment on training in the UK. Frontline Gastroenterol 2017;8(2):104–9.

37. Duloy A, Kaltenbach TR, Wood M, et al. Mo1709 a colon polypectomy report card improves polypectomy competency: results of a prospective quality improvement study. Gastrointest Endosc 2018;87(6):AB489.

38. Ansell J, Hurley JJ, Horwood J, et al. The Welsh Institute for Minimal Access Therapy colonoscopy suitcase has construct and concurrent validity for colonoscopic polypectomy skills training: a prospective, cross-sectional study. Gastrointest Endosc 2014;79(3):490–7.

39. Ansell J, Hurley JJ, Horwood J, et al. Can endoscopists accurately self-assess performance during simulated colonoscopic polypectomy? A prospective, cross-sectional study. Am J Surg 2014;207(1):32–8.

40. Jirapinyo P, Kumar N, Thompson CC. Validation of an endoscopic part-task training box as a skill assessment tool. Gastrointest Endosc 2015;81(4): 967–73.
41. Haycock AV, Youd P, Bassett P, et al. Simulator training improves practical skills in therapeutic GI endoscopy: results from a randomized, blinded, controlled study. Gastrointest Endosc 2009;70(5):835–45.

Best Practices for Resection of Diminutive and Small Polyps in the Colorectum

Douglas K. Rex, MD

KEYWORDS

- Diminutive polyp • Small polyp • Adenoma • Colonoscopy • Biopsy • Cold snare
- Electrocautery

KEY POINTS

- Most sessile or flat colorectal polyps less than 10 mm in size should be removed by cold snaring.
- Cold snaring is as effective or nearly as effective as hot snaring for lesions less than 10 mm in size and is safer and more efficient.
- Cold forceps are acceptable for 1- to 3-mm polyps provided there is no piecemealing.
- If cold forceps are used to remove 1- to 3-mm polyps, larger forceps are more effective than standard size forceps.
- Hot forceps have no role in the removal of polyps less than 10 mm in size.

INTRODUCTION

The optimal management of diminutive (1–5 mm) and small (6–9 mm) colorectal lesions is not a trivial matter for several reasons. First, the great majority (85%–90%) of all colorectal lesions are less than 10 mm in size. Therefore, the cost of resection in terms of polypectomy and pathology charges is substantial. In the United States alone, the pathology charges for these lesions exceeds $1 billion per year.[1] The risk of cancer in 1- to 5-mm lesions is negligible,[2] and in modern studies the risk in 6- to 9-mm lesions is less than 1%.[2] The risk of cancer in lesions less than 10 mm seems to decrease steadily in publications over time, probably reflecting the increasing resolution and detection afforded by high-definition colonoscopes.[2] Consistent with this observation, the prevalence of precancerous lesions is

Disclosure Statement: Consultant: Olympus Corporation, Boston Scientific, Medtronic, Aries, Braintree. Research Support: EndoAid, Olympus Corporation, Medivators. Ownership: Satisfai Health.
Division of Gastroenterology and Hepatology, Indiana University School of Medicine, Indiana University Hospital, 550 North University Boulevard, Suite 4100, Indianapolis, IN 46202, USA
E-mail address: drex@iu.edu

Gastrointest Endoscopy Clin N Am 29 (2019) 603–612
https://doi.org/10.1016/j.giec.2019.06.004
giendo.theclinics.com

about 50% for conventional adenomas and perhaps 8% to 10% for sessile serrated polyps (SSPs).[3–5] Collectively, this prevalence far exceeds the lifetime incidence of colorectal cancer, which is about 5% to 6% for persons reaching the age of 50 years. Thus, it seems important to use the safest methodology that maintains efficacy for this enormous number of lesions less than 10 mm in size that are overwhelmingly destined to never actually harm patients. Even though the per polyp risk of resection is considerably lower than for larger lesions, the absolute number of complications resulting from resection of lesions less than 10 mm can exceed the number from larger lesions within an endoscopy practice, solely because the smaller lesions are so much more numerous.[6] Finally, resecting all these small lesions has a significant impact on the efficiency of colonoscopy. Busy colonoscopists trying to maximize their efficiency are interested in what is the quickest way to achieve effective and safe resection.

LESION ASSESSMENT AND DOCUMENTATION

Modern colonoscopes allow for the accurate prediction of about 80% of diminutive as belonging to the conventional adenoma class versus the serrated class (hyperplastic polyps [HPs] and SSPs).[6] There is considerable value that extends to polyps less than 10 mm in size in learning to accurately apply a classification scheme such as the Narrow band imaging International Colorectal Endoscopic (NICE) classification developed for Olympus[7] (Olympus Corp, Center Valley, PA) or the BLI Adenoma Serrated International Classification developed for use with the Fuji 700 series using Blue Light Imaging[8] (Fujifilm, Valhalla, NY). The value extends beyond the "resect and discard" concept, which is well-established as effective, especially for narrow band imaging (NBI),[9] but which in daily practice encounters obstacles based on institutional rules regarding submitting resected tissue for pathologic evaluation, and financial incentives that are not aligned with the resect and discard paradigm.

The first use to put real-time polyp histology prediction to is the issue of whether to resect diminutive lesions or leave them in place.[10] The usual dogma is to resect conventional adenomas anywhere they occur in the colon. In addition, SSPs are considered neoplastic and should be resected whereas diminutive HPs are generally considered to not be premalignant and can be left in place. The NICE classification is concerned with pit and vessel patterns on the surface of lesions. As such, the only element in the NICE classification that concerns differentiation of SSPs from HPs is the occurrence of large open pits in SSPs.[11] The Workgroup on serrated polypS and Polyposis (WASP) classification incorporates gross morphologic features, including irregular surface, cloudlike features, and indistinct edges in addition to large open pits to distinguish SSP from HP.[11] However, it is not yet clear that the WASP criteria can be applied effectively to distinguish SSP from HP when the lesion size is 1 to 5 mm. Because the risk in NICE type 1 lesions in the proximal colon of being SSPs is substantial, NICE type 1 lesions in the proximal colon should generally be resected and submitted to pathology. In the rectosigmoid colon, however, the fraction of NICE type 1 lesions 1-5 mm in size that are SSPs is less than 2%.[12] Stated differently, the negative predictive value of NICE type 1 features for both adenoma and SSP is extremely high, and diminutive lesions in the rectosigmoid that have NICE type 1 features can be left in place without resection.

This author's practice is to resect all rectosigmoid lesions greater than 5 mm in size and to resect all diminutive rectosigmoid lesions that seem to be adenomas when examined in NBI or that seem to be NICE type 1 in NBI but have large open pits and therefore might be one of the uncommon rectosigmoid SSPs.

Finally, I tend to document each lesion that is resected with photography in NBI, unless the number of lesions makes this impractical. Part of the rationale is that 1- to 3-mm lesions that seems to very clearly be high confidence adenomas in NBI are read by our pathologists as normal tissue in about 15% of cases.[13] This finding is true regardless of whether the lesions are resected by snaring or forceps.[13] This phenomenon has been observed previously, and can be partly corrected by taking additional cuts through the formalin block storing the polyp.[14] However, it is only partially corrected by routine recuts, and the cause of the remaining failures to demonstrate adenoma pathologically is uncertain. Fragmentation of the specimen (resulting in capture of a tissue fragment that does not include the polyp) may partly account.[15] In any case, if the recuts do not show adenoma in a lesion that is clearly demonstrated in the photographs, I base the recommended on surveillance interval after including the lesion as an adenoma. Whether tiny adenomas really affect the subsequent risk of advanced lesions being identified is uncertain and arguable, but also a separate issue. The lesions are almost certainly real adenomas, given that they are identified at times on recuts and endoscopically they are indistinguishable from lesions that are proven pathologically to be adenomas.[13]

OPTIMAL RESECTION METHODS FOR DIMINUTIVE (1–5 MM) LESIONS

Randomized, controlled trials that have compared cold forceps with cold snaring consistently demonstrate that, when the polyp size increases to 4 mm, cold forceps resection becomes less effective than cold snaring.[16–18] The reason is almost certainly that removal of polyps 4 mm or greater in size using cold forceps requires piecemealing. Piecemealing in general is associated with higher recurrence rates than en bloc resection. In the case of cold forceps, the combination of bleeding and tissue disruption induced by the first bit almost certainly prevents accurate recognition and removal of any residual polyp. In addition, cold snaring is more efficient than cold forceps when polyp size increases to 4 mm, because resection in 1 piece using a snare is faster than taking multiple bits, particularly if the forceps have to be removed to empty tissue into a formalin container and then reintroduced into the colon.

Many experts (myself included) advocate using cold snaring for lesions more than 2 mm in size,[19] because even 3-mm lesions seem at times to require piecemealing (**Figs. 1** and **2**). Indeed, cold forceps are often used only to remove 1- to 2-mm polyps that are difficult to position in the 5 or 6 o'clock position. When cold forceps are used, it is clear that the larger the forceps the more effective the resection.[20,21] However, virtually the entire set of lesions 1 to 5 mm in size is removed by cold snaring when they can be positioned properly in the endoscopic field of view.

In 1992, the American Society for Gastrointestinal Endoscopy issued a document on proper usage of hot biopsy forceps.[22] The document endorsed hot forceps resection as an option for diminutive polyps only, and has not been updated since 1992. However, hot forceps have been shown to have substantial rates of ineffective resection, 17% and 53% in 2 studies.[23,24] Further, they are associated with a risk of delayed hemorrhage related to thermal injury and rarely have been associated with perforation.[25] Hot forceps result in thermal injury to deeper layers of the bowel wall in animal studies.[26] Relative to cold techniques, hot forceps resection of diminutive polyps results in severe injury to resected specimens, which can compromise pathologic assessment.[24] Given the efficacy of cold resection techniques for diminutive polyps, hot forceps are no longer appropriate for and have no role in the resection of diminutive polyps. The only remaining roles for hot forceps are in so-called hot avulsion, a technique used to salvage endoscopic mucosal resection (EMR) when snaring is not feasible because of very flat or fibrotic residual polyp.[27–29]

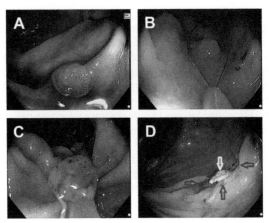

Fig. 1. Cold snaring of a 3-mm adenoma. (*A*) Lesion in NBI demonstrates pit and vessel pattern of a conventional adenoma. (*B*) Lesion seen in white light with the snare placed accurately before closure. (*C*) After resection without tenting the lesion stays on the resection site. (*D*) After retrieval of the specimen, the site inspection shows no residual polyp (*red arrows* point to the resection margin; *yellow arrow* points to the submucosal cord).

OPTIMAL RESECTION METHODS FOR SMALL (6–9 MM) LESIONS

A survey of US gastroenterologists in 2004 showed that cold and hot snaring were used almost equally by gastroenterologists to resect 4- to 6-mm polyps, but that hot snaring dominated the resection of 7- to 9-mm polyps.[30] Since then, randomized controlled trials have shown that cold snaring is as effective as hot snaring for 6- to 9-mm polyps.[31,32] Because the risk of hot snaring has been established as greater than cold snaring in randomized controlled trials performed in patients requiring

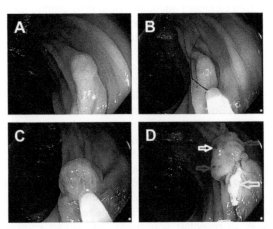

Fig. 2. Cold snaring of a 5-mm serrated lesion. (*A*) The lesion positioned at 5 o'clock in the endoscopic field before resection. (*B*) The snare placed accurately before closure. (*C*) The snare closed on the lesion with a rim of normal tissue around the polyp. (*D*) The transected specimen is seen above the defect. The white arrow points to the polyp. The red arrows point to the rim of normal tissue on the specimen around the polyp. The yellow arrow points to the submucosal cord created by transection.

reanticoagulation,[33] and comparisons of complication rates of hot and cold snaring using historical controls show that hot snaring causes more complications,[34] cold snaring is now the approach of choice to 6- to 9-mm sessile or flat polyps. In a large randomized controlled trial comparing hot with cold snaring for 4- to 9-mm polyps, cold snaring was as effective as hot snaring, and posttreatment hemorrhage requiring treatment occurred only in the hot snaring group.[31]

In a study comparing histologic specimens from cold and hot snaring, cold snaring resulted in muscularis mucosa in the specimen as often as hot snaring.[35] This observation seems to explain the equal effectiveness of hot and cold snaring. Hot snaring was found to extend into the deep submucosa in 60% of resections and to the muscularis propria in 20%.[36] Cold resections were limited to the shallow submucosa.[36] This finding could explain the likely increased risk of delayed hemorrhage with hot snaring, because a deeper injury would result in damage to the larger submucosal vessels. Other studies have found that histologic analysis of resected specimens shows more complete resection after hot snaring. In 1 study, complete resection was defined as removal in 1 piece, and normal resection margins were seen histologically.[37] The histologically defined complete resection rate for diminutive lesions was similar for hot and cold snaring, but for lesions 6 mm or greater the complete resection rate was 69.0% versus 43.5% with cold snaring ($P<.001$). Another study found that the entire muscularis mucosa could not be histologically defined in 21% of cold resection specimens.[38] Despite these concerning findings in histologic studies, clinical trials assessing the incidence of residual tissue on the resection site indicate cold snaring is as effective as hot snaring for lesions less than 10 mm in size. Mucosal defects after hot and cold snaring were compared immediately after resection and by repeat endoscopy 1 day later.[35] The mucosal defects with cold snaring were significantly larger than hot snaring defects immediately after resection. One day later the defect size had increased in diameter by 29% after hot snaring and decreased by 25% after cold snaring. The safety of the cold snare has allowed its extension to effective clearing of hundreds of polyps in familial adenomatous polyposis without a risk of complication.[39]

Randomized controlled trials have also included arms of EMR to standard hot or cold snaring for 6- to 9-mm polyps.[40] Thus far, EMR has not contributed dramatically or consistently to the efficacy of resection.[40] Because EMR is considerably less efficient than cold snaring because of the need to prepare and submucosally inject fluid, as well as the cost of the injection catheter, there is currently no strong rationale to use EMR in the resection of lesions less than 10 mm in the absence of endoscopic features suggesting advanced histology.

Cold snaring has been found twice to improve colonoscopy efficiency compared with hot snaring, presumably because there is no time required for the setup of a grounding pad, connecting the snare to the electrocautery source, and adjusting the electrocautery settings as needed. These studies suggested a 6-minute or approximately 25% decrease in total procedural time with cold versus hot snaring.[41,42] This effect almost certainly depends on how individual endoscopy centers manage the devices and materials needed to perform electrocautery. Two metaanalyses of cold versus hot snaring for colorectal lesions up to 10 mm in size concluded there was equal efficacy for the 2 techniques; however, cold snaring was more efficient and was associated with a trend toward less delayed hemorrhage.[43,44]

More data are needed regarding whether cold snaring can also be used for pedunculated lesions of less than 10 mm in size. My own anecdotal experience is that the technique is safe, although typically associated with more immediate bleeding than cold snare resection of flat or sessile lesions. I typically cold snare resect small pedunculated lesions with a thicker braided snare, which seems to crush small vessels more and be associated with less immediate bleeding. I prefer to snare these lesions below the stalk on through the normal mucosa adjacent to the polyp, and then vigorously wash the site with the colonoscope water jet to force fluid into the submucosa and tamponade small vessels. Each of these steps decreases immediate bleeding in my experience.

OTHER CONSIDERATIONS IN COLD SNARING
Technical Performance of Cold Snaring

The basic principles of optimal polypectomy technique for lesions less than 10 mm in size are encapsulated in the Direct Observation of Polypectomy Skills criteria[45] and covered in detail in Chapter 2. Stated briefly, the basic tenets are assessment of the lesion surface, rotation of the colonoscope so that the lesion is in the best position for snaring (**Fig. 3**), careful assessment of the entire surface of the lesion, maintaining the optimal distance from the lesion during snaring, accurate placement of the snare, retrieval of the lesion, and washing and inspecting the polypectomy defect for residual polyp[46] (see **Fig. 3**). The primary goal in cold snaring should be to keep the entire snare away from the border of the polyp, so that a rim of normal tissue one to several mm in width is transected circumferentially along with the polyp. In many cases of properly performed cold snare resections, the specimen is seen lying in the colon next to the mucosal defect, with the polyp entirely surrounded by normal mucosa on the specimen.

Specialized Cold Snares

The Exacto snare (US Endoscopy, Mentor, OH) and the Cold Captivator (Boston Scientific, MA) are small diameter, thin-wired, braided snares made specifically for cold snaring (**Fig. 4**). Randomized controlled trials have produced mixed results as to whether these specialized snares result in better resection efficacy compared with standard nonspecialized snares.[47,48] In 1 study of 8- to 10-mm polyps, the Exacto

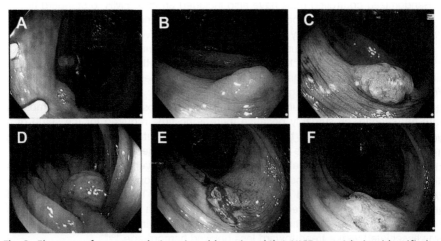

Fig. 3. Elements of proper technique in cold snaring. (A) A NICE type 1 lesion identified at the 7 o'clock position in the endoscopic field. (B) The lesion is rotated to the 5 o'clock position. (C) The lesion is fully inspected and characterized—in the case using NBI and -optical magnification. (D) The captured lesion including normal tissue surrounding the lesion. (E) The site after transection. (F) The site after washing and inspection.

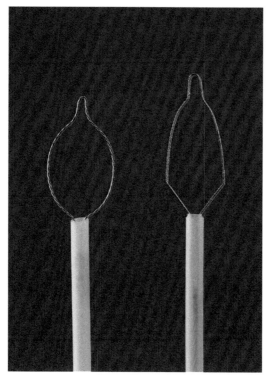

Fig. 4. Commercially available specialized cold snare. Left, Boston Scientific Cold Cap snare. Right, US Endoscopy Exacto. ([Left] *Courtesy of* Boston Scientific, Inc., Marlborough, MA; and [Right] *Courtesy of* US Endoscopy US. Unauthorized use not permitted.)

produced an 83% rate of complete resection compared with a standard snare.[47] In another study there was no difference.[48] Although the thinner wire in these snares results in easier tissue cutting than occurs with standard snares, additional study is needed to prove benefits compared with standard snares.

Submucosal Cords

After cold snaring the submucosal defect often seems to have a protruding white cord of tissue (see **Figs. 1** and **2**). This tissue is more commonly seen after ensnaring a larger polyp or a larger margin around a smaller polyp. When a larger surface is ensnared, the submucosa becomes entrapped in the snare and the snare often feels impacted on this tissue as the snare closes tightly. Pulling the tissue against the colonoscope tip and forcibly pulling the snare through the tissue is particularly likely to leave a white cord, because the snare closes on the submucosa and shapes and pulls the submucosa into a cord as the mucosa is stripped off. Two studies report that biopsies of this cord demonstrate only submucosa or muscularis mucosa and never residual polyp[49] or rarely residual polyp.[43] Thus, when the cord is present it can be left alone without further treatment or sampling.

In my experience it is safe to mechanically pull the snare through a larger piece of tissue. If force does not work, the snare can be reopened and smaller portions of the originally grasped mucosa can be taken and stripped off the submucosa.

ACKNOWLEDGMENTS

Ths work was supported by a gift gtom Scott Schurz and his children to the Indian University Foundation in the name of Douglas K. Rex.

REFERENCES

1. Kessler WR, Imperiale TF, Klein RW, et al. A quantitative assessment of the risks and cost savings of forgoing histologic examination of diminutive polyps. Endoscopy 2011;43:683–91.
2. Ponugoti PL, Cummings OW, Rex DK. Risk of cancer in small and diminutive colorectal polyps. Dig Liver Dis 2017;49:34–7.
3. Rex DK, Helbig CC. High yields of small and flat adenomas with high-definition colonoscopes using either white light or narrow band imaging. Gastroenterology 2007;133:42–7.
4. Abdeljawad K, Vemulapalli KC, Kahi CJ, et al. Sessile serrated polyp prevalence determined by a colonoscopist with a high lesion detection rate and an experienced pathologist. Gastrointest Endosc 2015;81:517–24.
5. JE IJ, de Wit K, van der Vlugt M, et al. Prevalence, distribution and risk of sessile serrated adenomas/polyps at a center with a high adenoma detection rate and experienced pathologists. Endoscopy 2016;48:740–6.
6. Kaltenbach T, Rastogi A, Rouse RV, et al. Real-time optical diagnosis for diminutive colorectal polyps using narrow-band imaging: the VALID randomised clinical trial. Gut 2015;64:1569–77.
7. Hewett DG, Kaltenbach T, Sano Y, et al. Validation of a simple classification system for endoscopic diagnosis of small colorectal polyps using narrow-band imaging. Gastroenterology 2012;143:599–607 e1.
8. Bisschops R, Hassan C, Bhandari P, et al. BASIC (BLI Adenoma Serrated International Classification) classification for colorectal polyp characterization with blue light imaging. Endoscopy 2018;50:211–20.
9. Committee AT, Abu Dayyeh BK, Thosani N, et al. ASGE Technology Committee systematic review and meta-analysis assessing the ASGE PIVI thresholds for adopting real-time endoscopic assessment of the histology of diminutive colorectal polyps. Gastrointest Endosc 2015;81:502.e1–16.
10. Rex DK, Kahi C, O'Brien M, et al. The American Society for Gastrointestinal Endoscopy PIVI (Preservation and Incorporation of Valuable Endoscopic Innovations) on real-time endoscopic assessment of the histology of diminutive colorectal polyps. Gastrointest Endosc 2011;73:419–22.
11. IJspeert JE, Bastiaansen BA, van Leerdam ME, et al. Dutch Workgroup serrated polypS & Polyposis (WASP). Development and validation of the WASP classification system for optical diagnosis of adenomas, hyperplastic polyps and sessile serrated adenomas/polyps. Gastroenterology 2016;65:963–70.
12. Ponugoti P, Lin J, Odze R, et al. Prevalence of sessile serrated adenoma/polyp in hyperplastic-appearing diminutive rectosigmoid polyps. Gastrointest Endosc 2017;85:622–7.
13. Ponugoti P, Rastogi A, Kaltenbach T, et al. Disagreement between high confidence endoscopic adenoma prediction and histopathological diagnosis in colonic lesions ≤ 3mm in size. Endoscopy 2019;51(3):221–6.
14. Rex DK. Narrow-band imaging without optical magnification for histologic analysis of colorectal polyps. Gastroenterology 2009;136:1174–81.
15. Barge W, Kumar D, Giusto D, et al. Alternative approaches to polyp extraction in colonoscopy: a proof of principle study. Gastrointest Endosc 2018;88:536–41.

16. Lee CK, Shim JJ, Jang JY. Cold snare polypectomy vs. Cold forceps polypectomy using double-biopsy technique for removal of diminutive colorectal polyps: a prospective randomized study. Am J Gastroenterol 2013;108:1593–600.

17. Kim JS, Lee BI, Choi H, et al. Cold snare polypectomy versus cold forceps polypectomy for diminutive and small colorectal polyps: a randomized controlled trial. Gastrointest Endosc 2015;81:741–7.

18. Park SK, Ko BM, Han JP, et al. A prospective randomized comparative study of cold forceps polypectomy by using narrow-band imaging endoscopy versus cold snare polypectomy in patients with diminutive colorectal polyps. Gastrointest Endosc 2016;83:527–32.e1.

19. Rex DK, Dekker E. How we resect colorectal polyps <20 mm in size. Gastrointest Endosc 2019;89(3):449–52.

20. Draganov PV, Chang MN, Alkhasawneh A, et al. Randomized, controlled trial of standard, large-capacity versus jumbo biopsy forceps for polypectomy of small, sessile, colorectal polyps. Gastrointest Endosc 2012;75:118–26.

21. Aslan F, Cekic C, Camci M, et al. What is the most accurate method for the treatment of diminutive colonic polyps? Standard versus jumbo forceps polypectomy. Medicine (Baltimore) 2015;94:e621.

22. Gilbert DA, DiMarino AJ, Jensen DM, et al. Status evaluation: hot biopsy forceps. American Society for Gastrointestinal Endoscopy. Technology Assessment Committee. Gastrointest Endosc 1992;38:753–6.

23. Peluso F, Goldner F. Follow-up of hot biopsy forceps treatment of diminutive colonic polyps. Gastrointest Endosc 1991;37:604–6.

24. Komeda Y, Kashida H, Sakurai T, et al. Removal of diminutive colorectal polyps: a prospective randomized clinical trial between cold snare polypectomy and hot forceps biopsy. World J Gastroenterol 2017;23:328–35.

25. Weston AP, Campbell DR. Diminutive colonic polyps: histopathology, spatial distribution, concomitant significant lesions, and treatment complications. Am J Gastroenterol 1995;90:24–8.

26. Metz AJ, Moss A, McLeod D, et al. A blinded comparison of the safety and efficacy of hot biopsy forceps electrocauterization and conventional snare polypectomy for diminutive colonic polypectomy in a porcine model. Gastrointest Endosc 2013;77:484–90.

27. Andrawes S, Haber G. Avulsion: a novel technique to achieve complete resection of difficult colon polyps. Gastrointest Endosc 2014;80:167–8.

28. Bassan MS, Cirocco M, Kandel G, et al. A second chance at EMR: the avulsion technique to complete resection within areas of submucosal fibrosis. Gastrointest Endosc 2015;81:757.

29. Kumar V, Broadley H, Rex DK. Safety and efficacy of hot avulsion as an adjunct to endoscopic mucosal resection (with videos). Gastrointest Endosc 2019;89(5):999–1004.

30. Singh N, Harrison M, Rex DK. A survey of colonoscopic polypectomy practices among clinical gastroenterologists. Gastrointest Endosc 2004;99:414–8.

31. Kawamura T, Takeuchi Y, Asai S, et al. A comparison of the resection rate for cold and hot snare polypectomy for 4-9 mm colorectal polyps: a multicentre randomised controlled trial (CRESCENT study). Gut 2018;67:1950–7.

32. Aslan F, Alper E, Vatansever S, et al. Tu1496 Cold SNARE polypectomy versus standard SNARE polypectomy in endoscopic treatment of small polyps. Gastrointest Endosc 2013;77:AB561.

33. Horiuchi A, Nakayama Y, Kajiyama M, et al. Removal of small colorectal polyps in anticoagulated patients: a prospective randomized comparison of cold snare and conventional polypectomy. Gastrointest Endosc 2014;79:417–23.

34. Yamashina T, Fukuhara M, Maruo T, et al. Cold snare polypectomy reduced delayed postpolypectomy bleeding compared with conventional hot polypectomy: a propensity score-matching analysis. Endosc Int Open 2017;05:E587–94.

35. Suzuki S, Gotoda T, Kusano C, et al. Width and depth of resection for small colorectal polyps: hot versus cold snare polypectomy. Gastrointest Endosc 2018;87:1095–103.

36. Takayanagi D, Nemoto D, Isohata N, et al. Histological comparison of cold versus hot snare resections of the colorectal mucosa. Dis Colon Rectum 2018;61:964–70.

37. Yamamoto T, Suzuki S, Kusano C, et al. Histological outcomes between hot and cold snare polypectomy for small colorectal polyps. Saudi J Gastroenterol 2017;23:246–52.

38. Shimodate Y, Itakura J, Mizuno M, et al. Factors associated with possibly inappropriate histological evaluation of excised specimens in cold-snare polypectomy for small colorectal polyps. J Gastrointest Liver Dis 2018;27:25–30.

39. Patel NJ, Ponugoti PL, Rex DK. Cold snare polypectomy effectively reduces polyp burden in familial adenomatous polyposis. Endosc Int Open 2016;4:E472–4.

40. Zhang Q, Gao P, Han B, et al. Polypectomy for complete endoscopic resection of small colorectal polyps. Gastrointest Endosc 2018;87:733–40.

41. Paspatis GA, Tribonias G, Konstantinidis K, et al. A prospective randomized comparison of cold vs hot snare polypectomy in the occurrence of postpolypectomy bleeding in small colonic polyps. Colorectal Dis 2011;13:e345–8.

42. Ichise Y, Horiuchi A, Nakayama Y, et al. Prospective randomized comparison of cold snare polypectomy and conventional polypectomy for small colorectal polyps. Digestion 2011;84:78–81.

43. Shinozaki S, Kobayashi Y, Hayashi Y, et al. Efficacy and safety of cold versus hot snare polypectomy for resecting small colorectal polyps: systematic review and meta-analysis. Dig Endosc 2018;30:592–9.

44. Qu J, Jian H, Li L, et al. Effectiveness and safety of cold versus hot snare polypectomy: a meta-analysis. J Gastroenterol Hepatol 2019;34:49–58.

45. Gupta S, Anderson J, Bhandari P, et al. Development and validation of a novel method for assessing competency in polypectomy: direct observation of polypectomy skills. Gastrointest Endosc 2011;73:1232–9.e2.

46. Duloy AM, Kaltenbach TR, Keswani RN. Assessing colon polypectomy competency and its association with established quality metrics. Gastrointest Endosc 2018;87:635–44.

47. Horiuchi A, Hosoi K, Kajiyama M, et al. Prospective, randomized comparison of 2 methods of cold snare polypectomy for small colorectal polyps. Gastrointest Endosc 2015;82:686–92.

48. Dwyer J, Tan JC, Urquhart P, et al. Su1655 a prospective comparison of cold snare polypectomy using traditional or dedicated cold snares for the resection of small sessile colorectal polyps. Gastrointest Endosc 2016;83:AB381.

49. Tutticci N, Burgess NG, Pellise M, et al. Characterization and significance of protrusions in the mucosal defect after cold snare polypectomy. Gastrointest Endosc 2015;82:523–8.

Endoscopic Assessment of the Malignant Potential of the Nonpolypoid (Flat and Depressed) Colorectal Neoplasms

Thinking Fast, and Slow

Ravishankar Asokkumar, MD[a], Carmel Malvar, BA[b,c],
Tiffany Nguyen-Vu, BA[b,c], Silvia Sanduleanu, MD, PhD[d],
Tonya Kaltenbach, MD, MS[b,c,e], Roy Soetikno, MD, MS, MSM[e,f,*]

KEYWORDS

- Endoscopy • Optical diagnosis • Colorectal cancer • Endoscopy training
- Cololonoscopy

KEY POINTS

- Thinking fast (reflex) and slow (rational) forms the basis of human decision making.
- We acquire knowledge by rationalizing findings and, in turn, the gained knowledge enables us to perform most tasks by reflex and others by rationale.
- In endoscopy, we gain knowledge through the cases we encounter in the endoscopy unit, the didactic lectures we listen to, and the relevant literature we read.
- This learning process has been practiced for decades despite having high potential for adverse effects on patient safety and requiring a significant amount of time before endoscopists achieve competence and confidence.
- Additionally, the current endoscopy training methodology does not meet the learning traits, skills, and needs of the newer generation, the millennial gastroenterologists.

Common sense, insight, practice and knowledge are required.
—Robert V. Rouse, MD (1948–2018)

[a] Department of Gastroenterology and Hepatology, Singapore General Hospital, 1 Hospital Drive, Singapore 169608, Singapore; [b] Department of Gastroenterology, Veterans Affairs Medical Center, 4150 Clement Street, San Francisco, CA 94121, USA; [c] Department of Medicine, University of California, 500 Parnassus Avenue, San Francisco, CA 94143, USA; [d] Division of Gastroenterology and Hepatology, Maastricht University Medical Center, Maastricht, P. Debyelaan 25, Maastricht 6229 HX, The Netherlands; [e] Advanced Gastrointestinal Endoscopy, Mountain View, CA, USA; [f] University of Indonesia, Kampus Baru UI Depok, Jawa Barat, Jakarta 16424, Indonesia
* Corresponding author. Advanced GI Endoscopy, Mountain View, CA.
E-mail address: soetikno@earthlink.net

Gastrointest Endoscopy Clin N Am 29 (2019) 613–628
https://doi.org/10.1016/j.giec.2019.06.006
1052-5157/19/© 2019 Elsevier Inc. All rights reserved.

INTRODUCTION

Thinking fast (reflex) and slow (rational) form the basis of human decision making.[1] We acquire knowledge by rationalizing findings and, in turn, the gained knowledge enables us to perform most tasks by reflex and others by rationale. In endoscopy, we gain knowledge through the cases we encounter in the endoscopy unit, the didactic lectures we listen to, and the relevant literature we read. This learning process has been practiced for decades despite having high potential for adverse effects on patient safety and requiring a significant amount of time before endoscopists achieve competence and confidence.[2] Additionally, the current endoscopy training methodology does not meet the learning traits, skills, and needs of the newer generation, the millennial gastroenterologists.[3,4] One example observed from the slow learning process has been concerning: endoscopic resection of larger colorectal neoplasm is still not uniformly practiced in the United States. In fact, recent literature showed an increase in the number of surgeries performed to treat benign colorectal neoplasms.[5,6]

In this article, we provide information on the assessment of the malignant potential of colorectal neoplasms. We took a modern approach to the topic and integrated relevant information that aligns with our thinking process. We used the theory of thinking fast and slow by Daniel Kahneman, recipient of the Nobel Prize in Economic Sciences, of how humans form thoughts. By doing so, we hope that the learning process can be expedited and practiced immediately. We have classified the content into "reflex knowledge," the knowledge that the readers must initially rationalize and subsequently memorize, and "rational knowledge," the knowledge of the rules and criteria that the readers need to understand and be familiar with. We focus on the preresection assessment of nonpolypoid colorectal neoplasms and only briefly discuss the assessment of polypoid, sessile-serrated adenoma/polyp, or inflammatory bowel disease (IBD) dysplasia.

PRINCIPLES

Endoscopic resection must be performed as safely as possible. The risk of immediate or delayed bleeding, perforation, and local or distant recurrence must be kept at a low or negligible rate. To achieve this goal, endoscopists need to analyze and interpret the endoscopic features of lesions, understand the risk of lymph node metastasis, carefully select patients, consider their preferences, follow the accepted indication, and adopt standardized resection techniques.

To ensure the long-term safety of endoscopic resection, it is essential to understand the risks of lymph node metastasis in early colorectal cancer. In the United States, surgery is the standard treatment of any invasive cancer into the submucosa.[7] This practice is to ensure the removal of potential lymph node metastasis. In Japan, endoscopic resection is the standard treatment of some of these patients.[8,9] Japanese experts consider that lesions with well or moderately differentiated adenocarcinoma of the colon or rectum with an invasion depth into the submucosa of less than or equal to 1000 µm and without lymphovascular invasion are safely treated by endoscopic resection. Kitajima and colleagues[10] described the risk of lymph node metastasis in such lesions as 0%. We look at the data statistically. Our meta-analysis showed that the risk of lymph node metastasis in nonpolypoid early cancer, with similar features irrespective of tumor size, is up to 3.6% because the upper limit of 95% confidence interval is such.[11–13] Therefore, although curative endoscopic resection is achieved for most early cancers, there is no guarantee that the risk of lymph node metastasis will be zero.

Patients' comorbidities and age play an important role in patient selection. Colorectal neoplasms usually grow slowly before progressing to advanced cancers.[14] In elderly patients, the risk of mortality from advanced age and medical comorbidities may outweigh the benefit of any treatment of an early colorectal cancer. However, in other patients, when the comorbidities and possibility of developing metastasis are low, overcoming risks through endoscopic resection becomes a suitable alternative to surgery.[15,16] Conversely, in younger patients with early colorectal cancer, the goal of treatment is to achieve oncologic cure and prevent delayed recurrence or metastasis. Surgery may be preferred over endoscopic resection in such situations.

Patient preferences must be included in the decision-making process. For example, when deciding to resect early rectal cancer, patients may prefer endoscopic resection rather than surgery because of their views on the low quality of life after a colostomy.[17]

KNOWLEDGE FOR DECISION MAKING

The skills and knowledge required for endoscopy include at least the technical and cognitive aspects. We apply technical skills and cognitive knowledge either by reflex or by rationale (purposeful thinking). Unfortunately, it is difficult to describe what we think by reflex. Others believe that reflex thinking is innately present (ie, we are born with it) or it is common sense (ie, there is no need to teach it), thus it is not possible to teach. We believe that it is a false presumption to assume that most endoscopists have such knowledge innately. Recent publications in endoscopy training have described the need to deconstruct reflex thinking during training, whenever possible, either verbally or through conscious competent trainers who have explicit knowledge and can break down each element of reflex thinking.[2–4] In the following, we describe our reflexive and cognitive thinking when assessing the malignant potential of a colorectal lesion.

REFLEXIVE THINKING
The Technical Part of Reflexive Thinking

Let us consider what our hands do reflexively when we assess a lesion. The process begins as soon as we identify a lesion. To optimize the assessment, we choose an endoscope with superior image quality when possible and maintain a straight scope position during withdrawal. We view the lesion from long, short (standard), and close-up locations (**Fig. 1**). Each view provides different, but complementary information. In addition to using white light, in short and close-up view, we further assess the lesion with dye, equipment-based image enhancement, or a combination of both. On insufflation and desufflation of the lumen, we also document the findings by taking still images and videos.

Long view

In the long view, we obtain the overall image of the lesion. We derive information about the size, anatomic location, position (in the rectum: left, right, anterior, and posterior wall), relationship to the surrounding structures, and macroscopic appearance. We look for potentially concerning areas (discussed later in section on cognitive reflex knowledge) and begin to roughly estimate their malignant potential. Then, we plan our approach for resection.

Short view (standard view)

In short view, we examine the border and every segment of the lesion. When the border becomes indistinct, we trace the innominate grooves present in normal mucosa until it disappears in neoplastic tissue. We examine the entire surface looking for the presence of ulceration, depression, and areas with a loss of pattern. In a large

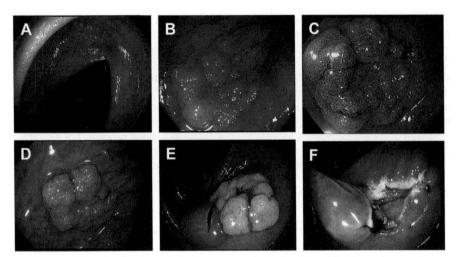

Fig. 1. The technical reflex knowledge. We assess the lesion from (*A*) a long view to characterize the morphology of the lesion, location on the bowel wall, and relationship to surrounding structures. (*B*) We then go closer and assess the lesion in short view. We look for the surface pattern and evaluate for abnormal signs. (*C*) After this, we assess the lesion in close-up view and use equipment-based image-enhanced endoscopy to study the vascular and surface pattern. (*D*) To discern the borders and pit pattern, we perform chromoendoscopy using diluted indigo carmine. (*E*) After establishing the suitability for resection, we perform endoscopic resection using the inject-and-cut endoscopic mucosal resection technique. We perform dynamic injection to elevate the lesion. (*F*) We apply blended current to resect the lesion en bloc whenever possible.

lesion, we examine the most proximal part of the lesion in a retroflex position when necessary.

Close-up view
Close-up view allows additional magnification of the surface pits and microvessels. We use the close-up view to confirm suspicious findings detected during the standard view assessment. Because of the limited optics of the standard colonoscopes, we use a distal attachment cap, which enhances image visualization and quality by stabilizing the focal length between the lesion and the lens. Additionally, the cap is helpful when imaging lesions that are located behind the mucosal folds.[18] Immersing the lesion under water can further magnify its surface patterns.

Use of image-enhanced endoscopy
We use equipment and dye-based image-enhanced endoscopy (IEE) reflexively. For most lesions less than 1 cm, narrow band imaging (NBI) or blue light imaging provides sufficient enhancement to learn the border, surface structure, and microvascular pattern. We use indigo carmine dye-based image enhancement to study the pit pattern, presence of depression, and borders of larger lesions. We train our assistants on dye preparation to hasten the chromoendoscopy process.

Insufflation and desufflation of the lumen
Gradually insufflating and desufflating the lumen provides detail on the pliability of the lesion. In advanced cancer, the lesion is firm, adherent, and fixated to the bowel wall. Deflation helps for better visualization of the lesion. For other lesions that flatten during

insufflation, deflation of the lumen creates an indentation within the lesion and allows easy recognition.

The Cognitive Part of Reflexive Thinking

Although we perform certain maneuvers reflexively, we think of certain findings reflexively. First, we use standardized nomenclature. We then call on a few key facts that we know extremely well. They are the memorized facts. We suggest readers become familiar with them.

Nomenclature

Standardized nomenclature is available for a clear and precise description of the neoplasm and its pathology by gastroenterologists, surgeons, pathologists, referring physicians, endoscopy nurses and technicians, and patients. The following terms are commonly used.[19,20]

Nonpolypoid colorectal neoplasms Nonpolypoid colorectal neoplasms include lesions with superficially elevated, flat, or depressed morphology. They are observed in approximately 10% of patients undergoing colonoscopy and are more likely to contain serious pathology (high-grade dysplasia or invasive carcinoma) compared with polypoid lesions of similar size.[21] The term "flat" lesions in clinical practice collectively represents neoplasms that are truly flat (in level with the surrounding mucosa), and those that are superficially elevated (slightly raised compared with normal surrounding mucosa). Because colorectal neoplasms that are truly flat are extremely rare except in patients with IBD, this colloquial definition of nonpolypoid colorectal neoplasms was made possible.

In patients with IBD, truly flat lesions are not uncommon; these neoplasms are often described as dysplasia. Thus, the SCENIC guidelines classified nonpolypoid colorectal dysplasias as flat, slightly elevated, and depressed (**Fig. 2**). In addition, the description of the lesion's border and presence of ulceration must be included.[22]

Lateral spreading tumors The term lateral spreading tumor (LST) is used to describe flat or superficial elevated lesions larger than 1 cm. LSTs are classified into two different types: the granular and the nongranular type.[23] The granular LST is further

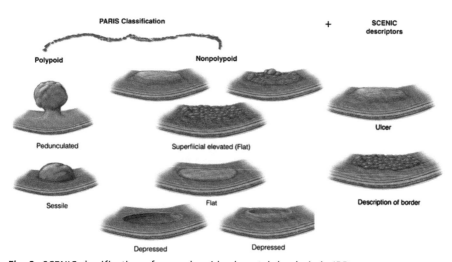

Fig. 2. SCENIC classification of nonpolypoid colorectal dysplasia in IBD.

subclassified into those with homogeneous granules and those with mixed nodules (**Fig. 3**). The nongranular LST is divided into two subtypes: flat elevated and pseudodepressed types (**Fig. 4**). Classifying the LSTs into different subtypes provides an estimate of the risk of invasion, potential location of the invasion, and possible difficulty with endoscopic resection.

Superficial versus deep lesion Superficial lesions are those that are believed to be endoscopically resectable, where the lesion can be "scooped out" using an endoscopic technique. Deep lesions are those that are deemed "too deep" to be scooped, and thus endoscopically unresectable (**Fig. 5**A, B).

Early versus advanced cancer Early cancer refers to cancer with the depth of invasion into the submucosa but not the deeper layers of the colon wall, irrespective of the status of the lymph nodes. Advanced cancer refers to invasion into the deeper layers, beyond the submucosa, with regional lymph node involvement or distant metastasis. Note that the term "early cancer" is often used to represent a superficial lesion and likewise, "deep lesion" is used for an advanced cancer. However, some clarity is required when using these terms synonymously because early cancers can either be superficial or deep, and deep lesions can be either early or advanced cancers (**Fig. 5**C).

First, the diagnosis of superficial and deep lesions is based on endoscopic assessment, whereas early and advanced cancers are diagnosed based on pathologic findings. Second, some early cancers on pathologic evaluation are confined to the superficial submucosa. These are categorized as superficial lesions and endoscopically resectable. Third, early cancer that extends into, but not beyond, the deep submucosa is classified as a deep lesion, and cannot be "scooped out" using endoscopy. Note that the term deep lesion here cannot be associated with advanced cancer because it does not extend to the muscular layer or serosa.

Depressed, pseudodepressed, and valley sign The terms depressed, pseudodepressed, and valley sign must be described accurately because they contain differential risks of submucosal invasion and thus varying levels of difficulty for endoscopic resection (**Fig. 6**).

Depressed neoplasms In a depressed neoplasm, a substantial portion of the lesion shows a significant decrease in height and a clear-cut indentation that can extend to a level below the adjacent normal mucosa. Depressed neoplasms have the highest risk

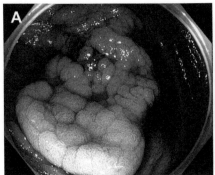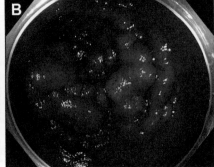

Fig. 3. Endoscopic image of a granular LST. (*A*) Homogeneous granular LST. (*B*) Mixed nodular LST.

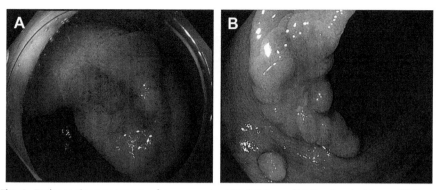

Fig. 4. Endoscopic appearance of nongranular LST. (*A*) Superficially elevated type. (*B*) Pseudodepressed type.

of submucosally invasive cancer and the risk increases with size.[24] Note that depressions are best appreciated using dye-based, rather than equipment-based, IEE because dye readily pools in the depressed area and enables accurate characterization.[25]

Pseudodepressed neoplasms In pseudodepressed neoplasms, there is no clear-cut depression. Instead, there is an inward slope of the surface with the deepest part

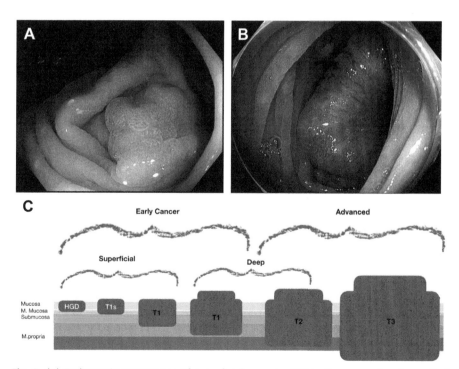

Fig. 5. (*A*) Endoscopic appearance of superficial granular LST in the appendiceal area that can be endoscopically removed. (*B*) A deep and advanced cancer that cannot be endoscopically resected. (*C*) Depth of invasion for superficial, deep, early, and advanced cancers.

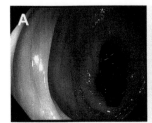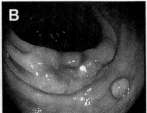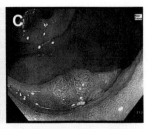

Fig. 6. (A) Depressed lesion characterized by a clear-cut indentation in the center of the lesion that extends to a level below the adjacent normal mucosa. (B) Pseudodepressed lesion characterized by inward slope of the surface. There are no hyperplastic changes at the edges. On chromoendoscopy, there is no pooling of dye in the center. (C) Valley sign typical of an adenoma characterized by dense capillary network at the center.

typically located at the center of the lesion. Pseudodepressed lesions also do not elicit a hyperplastic tissue change at the edges similar to depressed neoplasms. Thus, after dye spray, pseudodepressed neoplasms do not have a clear pooling of the dye. Of note, a pseudodepressed lesion has an increased risk of submucosal fibrosis and submucosal invasion.[26]

Valley sign The valley sign appears as a shallow slope with a dense capillary network in the center of a small adenoma. It is distinct from true depression and pseudodepression because the edges of the valley are sloping and do not extend to the level below normal mucosa. The valley sign has been validated as a marker of conventional adenomas, reaching a high specificity (91%) for adenoma in diminutive polyps.[27] Although small and diminutive adenomas are invariably benign, they should still be endoscopically resected thus making it important to recognize the valley sign.[27]

Facts used for reflex decision making
There are numerous "facts" that we use reflexively when assessing the malignant potential of a colorectal lesion. At times, a single fact is enough to diagnose submucosal invasive cancer. In other times, a single fact is not adequate and we need to combine two or more facts to make the diagnosis. Herein, we describe the facts that we must know when evaluating the malignant potential of colorectal neoplasms.

Depressed colorectal neoplasms Depressed lesions are believed to be biologically distinct: they grow rapidly into the bowel wall. Kudo and Kashida[24] showed that an 11- to 15-mm depressed lesion has a 70% chance of containing submucosally invasive cancer. The risk rapidly increases and reaches 87.5% for neoplasms greater than 20 mm in size. It is thus important to confirm the diagnosis of a depressed neoplasm using dye-based IEE.

Nongranular and large-nodular lateral spreading tumor Flat neoplasms larger than 1 cm are classified into four subtypes. This classification is imperative because each subtype has a different risk of submucosal invasion. Overall, the risk of submucosal invasion among the different LST subgroups ranges from low to intermediate.[12,28] In addition, each subtype has a specific location of where the invasion into the submucosa typically occurs. LST granular homogenous type has the lowest risk (<1%) of containing submucosal invasive cancer. The risk increases to 7.4% in LST granular with mixed nodules, and the submucosal invasion usually occurs beneath the largest nodule or the depressed portion **(Fig. 7)**.[28] Among LSTs, the LST nongranular with pseudodepression has the highest risk (26%) of harboring

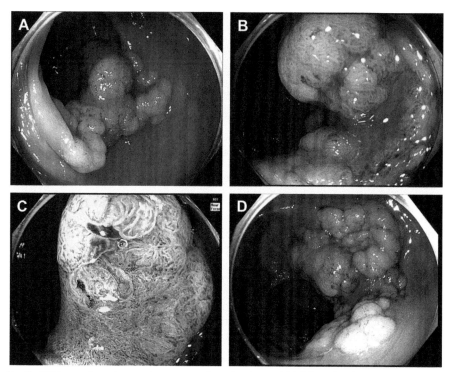

Fig. 7. (*A*) Long view shows a large granular mixed-type LST. (*B*) In the short view, a central depression is observed. (*C*) Equipment-based IEE assessment in the close-up view showed change in the surface and vascular pattern (NICE-III). (*D*) The lesion failed to lift at the center after injection suggesting submucosally invasive disease.

submucosal invasive cancer, especially in the pseudodepressed subgroup because it tends to have multiple foci of invasion.[28] Although they are biologically aggressive, LST nongranular with pseudodepression type lesions only account for 7% of all LSTs, whereas the other three subtypes each account for about 30% of LSTs.[28] To increase our specificity and diagnostic accuracy for detecting invasive cancer, we use image enhancement techniques to obtain additional supportive findings.

Fold convergence In superficial lesions, the neoplasm and the surrounding mucosa are pliable. Their shape is remodeled with air insufflation and desufflation. One of the characteristic findings of deep submuocsal invasion is the loss of this remodeling ability; they become firm and fixed to the bowel wall and the surrounding mucosa starts to converge toward the periphery of the lesion. Saitoh and colleagues[25] showed that converging folds frequently occur in deep submucosal invasion and is highly specific (93%) and predictive (89%) for advanced cancer.

In addition, the presence of color change, ulceration, spontaneous bleeding, surface irregularity, and the protrusion or overextension of the lesions suggests the presence of deep submucosal invasion.[26,29] In such cases, we perform image enhancement to increase our discriminative ability and to arrive at a diagnosis (**Fig. 8**).

Dye-based image-enhanced endoscopy: type V pit pattern Kudo and colleagues[29] showed, with the use of magnifying endoscopy, that the pit pattern changes based

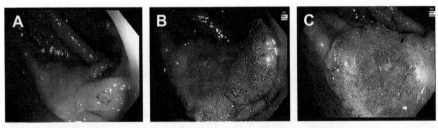

Fig. 8. Endoscopic appearance of fold convergence. (*A, B*) A depressed lesion with hyperplastic peripheral change is seen. The lesion fixated to the bowel wall and is firm in appearance. The mucosal folds are seen converging to the periphery of the lesion. (*C*) Equipment-based IEE showed distorted vascular and surface pattern confirming advanced disease.

on the degree of glandular proliferation within a neoplasm. In clinical practice, we use nonmagnifying dye-based chromoendoscopy using indigo carmine to assess the LST subtype and study the pit pattern of neoplasms because magnifying colonoscopes are not widely available.

The changes in the pit pattern are regular, irregular, or distorted. Invasive cancer usually presents with a distorted (type Vn) or irregular pit pattern with a demarcated area (type Vi). Matsuda and colleagues[30] showed that identification of invasive pit pattern is specific (99%) and is highly accurate (99%) in detecting an advanced cancer. We strongly recommend that the Kudo type Vi and Vn pattern be remembered and familiarized.

Equipment-based image-enhanced endoscopy: NICE III pattern Similar to pit pattern changes, the caliber and pattern of surface and submucosal microvessels transforms when the lesion progresses into cancer. These changes are better appreciated using equipment-based IEE. We use NBI technology without magnification because it is universally adopted in gastrointestinal practice.[31,32]

With NBI, the neoplasm is artificially classified into three groups using the NICE classification, which is based on color, vessel, and surface appearance. Among them, the type 3 group represents deep submucosal invasion, which presents irregular and disrupted vessels and amorphous or absent surface pattern. Puig and coworkers[33] have shown that recognition of the type 3 NICE pattern is highly specific (96%) and accurate (95%) for diagnosing advanced cancer, even when performed by nonexpert endoscopists. Thus, it should be memorized (**Fig. 9**).

Nonlifting sign We perform submucosal injection only after completing the previously described assessments. The lesion's response to submucosal injection may also serve as a diagnostic tool to detect invasive cancer. Kato and colleagues[34] classified the response to submucosal injection into four types: (1) complete smooth lifting where the lesion is stretched evenly; (2) complete hard lifting where the lesions lifts, but maintains its original shape and does not stretch; (3) incomplete/partial lifting where the surrounding mucosa lifts higher than the lesion; and (4) nonlifting where only the surrounding mucosa elevates after injection.

Nonlifting and incomplete lifting occurs when there is submucosal fibrosis or desmoplastic change from tumor invasion (see **Fig. 7**). Submucosal fibrosis, however, may also be a sequelae to a previous biopsy, polypectomy, or tattoo injection, and may falsely mimic the nonlifting sign. In such situations, nonlifting should be interpreted with caution. In the absence of previous therapy, Kobayashi and colleagues[35] showed that the nonlifting sign is highly specific (97%) and accurate (94%) for detecting invasive cancer in nonpolypoid colorectal neoplasms.

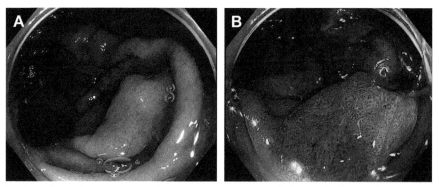

Fig. 9. Endoscopic appearance of NICE type 3 pit pattern. (*A*) A small, firm, adherent lesion that fails to flatten with insufflation is seen. (*B*) NBI evaluation showed irregular and disrupted vessels and area of absent surface pattern suggesting submucosally invasive cancer.

RATIONAL THINKING

Although we reflexively perform the procedure and think of the findings, our rational thinking, the "System 2" thinking, as Kahneman calls it, periodically performs checking to ensure that the maneuvers and decisions are correct. Our System 2 is also put into action when we are "stuck" (eg, we are unable to accurately determine if a lesion is submucosally invasive or not).

Technical Skills Available with Rational Thinking

We have used the following techniques to improve visualization: use of water immersion, use of antispasmodic, retroflexion viewing, and using dye-based IEE. Water immersion can help by inflating the lumen. As it is infused or sprayed, water not only cleans the surface, but can also open the crypts and separate the glands better because water allows them to be buoyed. Lesions tend to look better underwater. Note that there are no magnification changes. Occasionally, colon contractions prevent visualization. In such cases, we use antispasmodics, such as hyoscine butylbromide or glucagon. Retroflexion in the right colon or rectum, change of the patient's position, or abdominal pressure can also improve visualization. We also used indigo carmine to determine if the lesion has depressed area or not.

Cognitive Knowledge of Rational Thinking

Cognitively, we use the rules and the criteria as described previously, weigh the significance and implication of each positive finding, and consider patient preference in decision making. We may also use our prior knowledge from the experiences we have (**Fig. 10**).

Decision making is straight forward if the neoplasm displays a single or a combination of the specific findings of deep submucosal invasion, such as large depression, fold convergence, type Vn pit pattern, NICE III NBI pattern, or nonlifting sign.[36] Such cases should preferentially be referred for surgical resection. Difficulty arises when the signs are confusing. For example, when a lesion displays some signs that are type 2 and others that are type 3, then it is difficult to decide whether the lesion is type 2 or type 3. In these situations we need to adhere to the systematic examination process and carefully assess the lesion for the presence of specific high-risk features. Then, we combine findings from the different signs. When the lesion is determined to harbor submucosal invasion, surgical rather than endoscopic

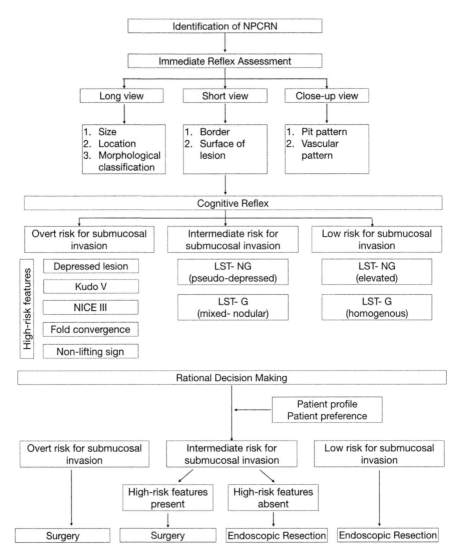

Fig. 10. Endoscopic assessment and decision-making framework for nonpolypoid colorectal neoplasm. G, granular; NG, nongranular; NPCRN, nonpolypoid colorectal neoplasm.

resection may be considered. In all other lesions with low-risk features, endoscopic resection is safely performed.

Decisions, however, can be skewed because of heuristics and biases. When answering basic and complex questions, our reflexes (System 1) rely on careful attention and draw information from one's memory to produce the answers. Our mind, by using System 1, tries to generate these answers with minimal intention or effort. However, our rationale (System 2) continuously checks System 1. When assessing the potential for invasive cancer, because we are not good at combining the different specificities, we reduce probabilities and predictive values to simpler basic assessments. We call these basic assessments heuristics. Although generally useful, these heuristics can give rise to systematic errors. When left unaddressed, these systematic errors (biases) may affect a physician's judgment or hinder their ability to make accurate diagnoses or treatment calls. Listed next are biases frequently encountered in endoscopy.

1. *Anchoring bias* is the tendency to rely too heavily on one trait or piece of information when making judgements/decisions. Anchors are hard to ignore, even when they are irrelevant. For example, a patient comes back because their previous colonoscopy was unsuccessful because of bad preparation. However, their last endoscopist reports seeing a lesion in the hepatic flexure. The physician then fixates on examining the hepatic flexure to locate this lesion while disregarding the importance of performing a thorough examination on the rest of the colon.
2. *Availability bias* is the tendency for recent or vivid events to affect the estimate of the probability the event will occur again. For example, a physician may encounter a cancerous lesion one day and find a large lesion in another patient the following day. Because the memory of finding the cancer is vivid, the physician is likely to overestimate the probability of the latter lesion being cancerous, despite that the incidence of cancerous lesions is low.
3. *Confirmation bias* is the tendency to search for information that confirms one's beliefs. For example, on detecting a lesion that is darker than the surrounding mucosa, the endoscopist forms the opinion that the polyp is type 2. He or she then performs closer inspection to answer the question *"is this a type 2 lesion?"* In doing so, the endoscopist limits themselves to only confirming that the lesion is indeed type 2 while unconsciously discounting that there are key features of a type 3 lesion also present.
4. *Status quo bias* is the preference for the current state of affairs, despite other better options being available. For instance, much data have shown that endoscopic techniques, such as endoscopic mucosal resection (EMR) and endoscopic submucosal dissection, are most effective for resecting large lesions. A practitioner, who encounters a large pseudodepressed LST, may choose to perform hot snare polypectomy over EMR, even though EMR is the most optimal resection method for this type of lesion. In this case, the status quo bias affected the practitioner because he or she chose to stick with the technique that he or she can easily perform, rather than the more challenging technique or referring the patient to another endoscopist.

When we assess whether a lesion is malignant or not, we should often consider if our assessment is biased or not. The consequences of these biases may be far reaching; they may compromise our ability to perform thorough examinations or to make the best diagnostic and treatment decisions. Although there is no one solution that can eliminate all of these biases, becoming more cognizant of the different kinds of biases that exist, and thus more aware of their presence, may help the endoscopist to address their biases. Furthermore, it is important to implement a system of constant feedback and self-assessment so that the endoscopist can reinforce good practices, reflect on their mistakes, and recalibrate their methods to become better.

SUMMARY

The assessment of malignant potential of colorectal neoplasms may be used more often when the required information is aligned with our thinking process. Rational decision making for the assessment of the malignant potential of a colorectal neoplasm is based on common sense, insight, knowledge, and practice rather than subjectivity, intuition, and personal preference. The systematic classification of the required knowledge in this article serves as a guide to enable physicians to understand the principles of endoscopic assessment.

ACKNOWLEDGMENTS

This article is dedicated to our pathologist, Robert Vance Rouse, MD, who made it possible for us to understand the flat and depressed colorectal neoplasms at the Veterans Affairs Palo Alto, CA. Without his willingness to have an open mind of the possible existence of the flat lesions among our patients and his dedication to study every early colorectal cancer we encountered, we would not have been able to write this article.

REFERENCES

1. Kahneman D. Thinking, fast and slow. New York: Farrar, Straus and Giroux; 2011.
2. Adler DG, Bakis G, Coyle WJ, et al. Principles of training in GI endoscopy. Gastrointest Endosc 2012;75(2):231–5.
3. Soetikno R, Kolb JM, Nguyen-Vu T, et al. Evolving endoscopy teaching in the era of the millennial trainee. Gastrointest Endosc 2019;89(5):1056–62.
4. Mahmood T, Scaffidi MA, Khan R, et al. Virtual reality simulation in endoscopy training: current evidence and future directions. World J Gastroenterol 2018; 24(48):5439–45.
5. Peery AF, Cools KS, Strassle PD, et al. Increasing rates of surgery for patients with nonmalignant colorectal polyps in the United States. Gastroenterology 2018;154(5):1352–60.e3.
6. Martin L, Yu JX, Gawron A, et al. Elective colectomy for the treatment of benign colon polyps: national surgical trends, outcomes and cost analysis: 98. Am J Gastroenterol 2017;112:S47–9.
7. Rex DK, Hassan C, Dewitt JM. Colorectal endoscopic submucosal dissection in the United States: why do we hear so much about it and do so little of it? Gastrointest Endosc 2017;85(3):554–8.
8. Watanabe T, Muro K, Ajioka Y, et al. Japanese Society for Cancer of the Colon and Rectum (JSCCR) guidelines 2016 for the treatment of colorectal cancer. Int J Clin Oncol 2018;23(1):1–34.
9. Bartel MJ, Brahmbhatt BS, Wallace MB. Management of colorectal T1 carcinoma treated by endoscopic resection from the Western perspective. Dig Endosc 2016;28(3):330–41.
10. Kitajima K, Fujimori T, Fujii S, et al. Correlations between lymph node metastasis and depth of submucosal invasion in submucosal invasive colorectal carcinoma: a Japanese collaborative study. J Gastroenterol 2004;39(6):534–43.
11. Kaltenbach T, Saito Y, Tada K, et al. Su1522 incidence of lymph node metastasis from sessile or nonpolypoid early colon cancer: stratified criteria to decide when to operate or when to watch. Gastrointest Endosc 2011;73(4). AB291–A292.
12. Bogie RMM, Veldman MHJ, Snijders L, et al. Endoscopic subtypes of colorectal laterally spreading tumors (LSTs) and the risk of submucosal invasion: a meta-analysis. Endoscopy 2018;50(3):263–82.
13. Mou S, Soetikno R, Shimoda T, et al. Pathologic predictive factors for lymph node metastasis in submucosal invasive (T1) colorectal cancer: a systematic review and meta-analysis. Surg Endosc 2013;27(8):2692–703.

14. Brenner H, Hoffmeister M, Stegmaier C, et al. Risk of progression of advanced adenomas to colorectal cancer by age and sex: estimates based on 840,149 screening colonoscopies. Gut 2007;56(11):1585–9.
15. Pontone S, Palma R, Panetta C, et al. Endoscopic mucosal resection in elderly patients. Aging Clin Exp Res 2017;29(Suppl 1):109–13.
16. Gaglia A, Skouras T, Bond A, et al. OC-070 Endoscopic mucosal resection in the elderly. Gut 2017;66(Suppl 2):A37–8.
17. Matsuoka H, Masaki T, Kobayashi T, et al. Which is the preference of choice either life with a stoma or evacuatory disorder following rectal cancer surgery? Hepato-gastroenterology 2011;58(107–108):749–51.
18. Sanchez-Yague A, Kaltenbach T, Yamamoto H, et al. The endoscopic cap that can (with videos). Gastrointest Endosc 2012;76(1):169–78.e1-2.
19. The Paris endoscopic classification of superficial neoplastic lesions: esophagus, stomach, and colon: November 30 to December 1, 2002. Gastrointest Endosc 2003;58(6 Suppl):S3–43.
20. Rex DK, Hassan C, Bourke MJ. The colonoscopist's guide to the vocabulary of colorectal neoplasia: histology, morphology, and management. Gastrointest Endosc 2017;86(2):253–63.
21. Soetikno RM, Kaltenbach T, Rouse RV, et al. Prevalence of nonpolypoid (flat and depressed) colorectal neoplasms in asymptomatic and symptomatic adults. JAMA 2008;299(9):1027–35.
22. Laine L, Kaltenbach T, Barkun A, et al. SCENIC international consensus statement on surveillance and management of dysplasia in inflammatory bowel disease. Gastrointest Endosc 2015;81(3):489–501.e26.
23. Kudo S, Lambert R, Allen JI, et al. Nonpolypoid neoplastic lesions of the colorectal mucosa. Gastrointest Endosc 2008;68(4 Suppl):S3–47.
24. Kudo SE, Kashida H. Flat and depressed lesions of the colorectum. Clin Gastroenterol Hepatol 2005;3(7 Suppl 1):S33–6.
25. Saitoh Y, Obara T, Watari J, et al. Invasion depth diagnosis of depressed type early colorectal cancers by combined use of videoendoscopy and chromoendoscopy. Gastrointest Endosc 1998;48(4):362–70.
26. Uraoka T, Saito Y, Matsuda T, et al. Endoscopic indications for endoscopic mucosal resection of laterally spreading tumours in the colorectum. Gut 2006; 55(11):1592–7.
27. Rex DK, Ponugoti P, Kahi C. The "valley sign" in small and diminutive adenomas: prevalence, interobserver agreement, and validation as an adenoma marker. Gastrointest Endosc 2017;85(3):614–21.
28. Yamada M, Saito Y, Sakamoto T, et al. Endoscopic predictors of deep submucosal invasion in colorectal laterally spreading tumors. Endoscopy 2016;48(5): 456–64.
29. Kudo S, Hirota S, Nakajima T, et al. Colorectal tumours and pit pattern. J Clin Pathol 1994;47(10):880–5.
30. Matsuda T, Fujii T, Saito Y, et al. Efficacy of the invasive/non-invasive pattern by magnifying chromoendoscopy to estimate the depth of invasion of early colorectal neoplasms. Am J Gastroenterol 2008;103(11):2700–6.
31. Hayashi N, Tanaka S, Hewett DG, et al. Endoscopic prediction of deep submucosal invasive carcinoma: validation of the narrow-band imaging international colorectal endoscopic (NICE) classification. Gastrointest Endosc 2013;78(4):625–32.
32. Hewett DG, Kaltenbach T, Sano Y, et al. Validation of a simple classification system for endoscopic diagnosis of small colorectal polyps using narrow-band imaging. Gastroenterology 2012;143(3):599–607.e1.

33. Puig I, Lopez-Ceron M, Arnau A, et al. Accuracy of the narrow-band imaging international colorectal endoscopic classification system in identification of deep invasion in colorectal polyps. Gastroenterology 2019;156(1):75–87.
34. Kato H, Haga S, Endo S, et al. Lifting of lesions during endoscopic mucosal resection (EMR) of early colorectal cancer: implications for the assessment of resectability. Endoscopy 2001;33(7):568–73.
35. Kobayashi N, Saito Y, Sano Y, et al. Determining the treatment strategy for colorectal neoplastic lesions: endoscopic assessment or the non-lifting sign for diagnosing invasion depth? Endoscopy 2007;39(8):701–5.
36. Burgess NG, Hourigan LF, Zanati SA, et al. Risk stratification for covert invasive cancer among patients referred for colonic endoscopic mucosal resection: a large multicenter cohort. Gastroenterology 2017;153(3):732–42.e1.

How to Perform Wide-Field Endoscopic Mucosal Resection and Follow-up Examinations

Michael J. Bourke, MBBS, FRACP[a,b,*], Bilel Jideh, BMedSci, MBBS, FRACP[a,b]

KEYWORDS

- Endoscopic mucosal resection • Laterally spreading lesion • Polyp
- Colorectal neoplasm • Colorectal cancer • Colonoscopy

KEY POINTS

- Wide-field endoscopic mucosal resection (EMR) is safe, effective, and superior to surgery for management of noninvasive laterally spreading colorectal lesions.
- Careful assessment of the lesion before resection provides essential information, including the risk of submucosal invasion.
- Adjuvant thermal ablation to the resection margin substantially reduces the risk of recurrent adenoma in long-term follow-up.
- The risk of recurrence can be predicted using the Sydney EMR Recurrence Tool.
- Recurrent adenoma can be accurately detected using standardized imaging of the post-EMR scar and effectively treated.

INTRODUCTION

Colorectal cancer (CRC) is a leading cause of cancer-related morbidity and mortality.[1] Most CRC arises from the well-described adenoma-to-carcinoma sequence.[2] Endoscopic resection of precancerous polyps has been shown to circumvent this pathway and reduce CRC incidence and mortality.[3–5]

Up to 90% of colonic polyps encountered during routine colonoscopy are less than 10 mm in size, do not contain advanced disease, and are easily excised by conventional snare polypectomy by appropriately trained colonoscopists.[6–8] A small proportion of colonic polyps are large, flat, or sessile lesions greater than 20 mm, collectively termed

Disclosure: Neither author received any funds related to this article. Neither author has any conflict of interests to declare.
[a] Department of Gastroenterology and Hepatology, Endoscopy Unit, Westmead Hospital, Cnr Hawkesbury & Darcy Roads, Westmead, Sydney, New South Wales 2145, Australia; [b] Westmead Clinical School, University of Sydney, Sydney, New South Wales, Australia
* Corresponding author. Suite 106a, 151-155 Hawkesbury Road, Westmead, Sydney, New South Wales, 2145, Australia
E-mail address: michael@citywestgastro.com.au

laterally spreading lesions (LSLs). These LSLs have a varied risk for submucosal invasion (SMI) and require advanced imaging and resection techniques to optimize outcomes.[9,10]

Wide-field endoscopic mucosal resection (WF-EMR) is the primary method for managing LSLs. Over the last decade the technique has been systematically studied and sequentially refined to emerge as a safe and highly effective technique for LSLs of all sizes.[11-15] Compared with surgical resection, endoscopic mucosal resection (EMR) has been shown to have superior clinical outcomes and substantially reduced health care costs.[16,17] Same-day discharge is possible in more than 95% of cases. This article outlines the current best-practice technique of WF-EMR and the associated follow-up examinations.

PREPARATION FOR WIDE-FIELD ENDOSCOPIC MUCOSAL RESECTION

Like all high-quality endoscopy, safe and successful EMR starts with careful preparation, which seems obvious but is often overlooked. Colonoscopists must know the patient well and be familiar with all the procedural components, including the available endoscopes, snares and ancillary devices, the electrosurgical generator, and the tools for managing adverse events. Good rapport with the nursing staff, the fellows (if any), and the sedationists is crucial. The EMR procedure is a team effort and all members must fulfill their roles while being cognizant of the various phases and dynamics of the procedure.

EQUIPMENT FOR WIDE-FIELD ENDOSCOPIC MUCOSAL RESECTION
Injection Solution

Submucosal injection is a core component of EMR. It expands the submucosal space and elevates the lesion away from the muscularis propria, thereby providing a safety cushion for snare excision of the lesion. Although saline is effective and widely available, colloid solutions have been shown to be superior. Succinylated gelatin (Gelofusion: Braun, Melsungen, Germany) is the colloid solution used in our unit. In a randomized trial it proved superior to normal saline, with significantly lower injections, fewer resections, and shorter procedure time.[18]

Inert dye (preferably indigo carmine) stains the submucosa and therefore provides helpful guidance for resection within the correct tissue plane; if the deeper nonstaining muscularis propria is entered, an obvious disruption of the stained tissue plane is noted.[10] The dye also defines the extent of the fluid cushion and the margin of the lesion, which is advantageous in subtle lesions.

Diluted epinephrine (1:10,000) is included in the injectate; it helps reduce intraprocedural bleeding to keep the field clear. In a large multicentre analysis of more than 2000 patients, it was also shown to reduce delayed bleeding.[19]

Snares

Snares are available in a range of sizes, wire diameters (0.28–0.5 mm), and configurations. Several different snares may be required during complex WF-EMR. Snare selection is an individual choice to some extent. Stiff snares are preferred because they provide better tissue capture. Thin wire snares (0.3–0.4 mm) may provide swifter and closer tissue transection, making evaluation of the defect margins for residual adenoma easier. Small, stiff, thin wire snares (wire diameter ≤ 30 mm) are precise and effective for small residual adenoma at the lesion margin.

Electrosurgical Generator

Microprocessor-controlled electrosurgical generators (VIO 300D: ERBE, Tübingen, Germany, ESG100; Olympus Medical, Tokyo, Japan) are most commonly used for

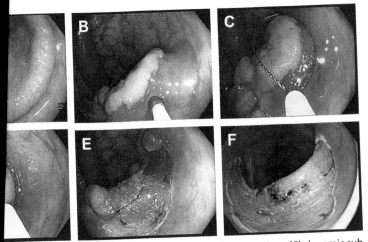

of a 40-mm Paris 0-IIa granular lesion. (A) Lesion overview, (B) dynamic sub-
n, (C) snare placement including 2 to 3 mm of normal mucosa, (D) tissue cap-
d submucosal tissue following resection, (F) completed tissue resection with
DMI.

rected by lifting the captured tissue into the lumen and slightly opening
are to release the deeper tissue and then closing again.
ansection of the ensnared tissue, which is usually achieved with 1 to 3
 of a microprocessor-controlled generator using fractionated current.
er transection phase raises concern for muscularis propria entrapment,
or invasive disease.
the mucosal defect after every resection for adequacy of resection, DMI
ed later), and for residual polyp. Irrigating into the defect (with either

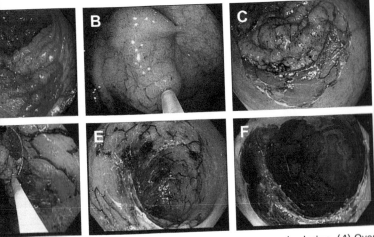

EMR of 100-mm focally circumferential Paris 0-IIa + Is granular lesion. (A) Over-
on, (B) dynamic submucosal injection, (C) exposed submucosal tissue, (D) snare
 retroflexed position, (E) completed tissue resection with no evidence of DMI,
t thermal ablation to the resection margin (discussed later).

WF-EMR. These processors deliver alternating cycles of high-frequency short-pulse
cutting with more prolonged coagulation current and adjust power output according
to the impedance signals received from the return electrode. Consequently, the risk
of unnecessary deep tissue injury is limited. The energy delivery is optimized to
achieve excision of the mucosal neoplasm.

LESION ASSESSMENT

Careful assessment of the lesion before resection is vital because it informs the risk of
SMI, submucosal scarring, and endoscopic accessibility. These aspects may
mandate an alternate management approach. Suspected superficial SMI may be suitable for endoscopic resection but this should be en bloc, so endoscopic submucosal
dissection (ESD) may be preferred or surgery may be more appropriate. Predicted
deep SMI is best managed by surgery.

Lesion assessment entails overview and focal interrogation components. In overview
Paris morphology and surface topography (granular, nongranular, or mixed) stratify
the risk of SMI.[11,20,21] For instance, a homogeneous Paris 0-IIa granular lesion has a
low risk of SMI at 1% to 2%, whereas a Paris 0-IIa + IIc nongranular lesion has the highest
risk of SMI of up to ~70% (**Fig. 1**).

Focal interrogation of areas at risk of SMI is essential. This interrogation may be
classified by the mucosal crypt orifices (the pit pattern) according to the Kudo

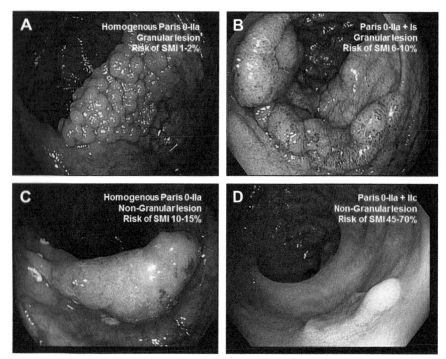

Fig. 1. Various types of LSL and corresponding risk of SMI. (*Data from* Moss A, Bourke MJ,
Williams SJ, Hourigan LF, Brown G, Tam W, et al. Endoscopic mucosal resection outcomes
and prediction of submucosal cancer from advanced colonic mucosal neoplasia. Gastroenterology 2011;140(7):1909–18; and Uraoka T, Saito Y, Matsuda T, Ikehara H, Gotoda T, Saito
D, et al. Endoscopic indications for endoscopic mucosal resection of laterally spreading tumours in the colorectum. Gut 2006;55(11):1592–70.)

classification,[22] the vascular pattern according to the Sano classification,[23] or more recently the Narrow-Band Imaging International Colorectal Endoscopic (NICE) classification.[24] These classification criteria can be used to predict histology and SMI.[11,24,25] Pit pattern types III and IV indicate benign adenoma, whereas pit pattern type V is associated with SMI.

A useful general principle is that a benign lesion has a homogeneous surface pit pattern without any obvious transition line or demarcation zone. SMI may be considered as overt or covert based on endoscopic imaging. A recent advance in lesion assessment is risk stratification for covert SMI; that is, the realization that certain gross LSL morphologies may be stratified for submucosal invasive cancer in the absence of highly suggestive surface endoscopic features, such as type V pit pattern. In a prospective study, the following features were associated with increased risk for covert malignancy: distal colon (rectosigmoid location), combined Paris classification (eg, 0-IIa + Is), nongranular surface topography, and increasing lesion size.[26] These new findings can be used to further rationalize which patients undergo EMR or ESD based on local expertise and resources, which is especially pertinent in the rectum, where endoscopic cure of low-risk submucosal cancer by en bloc R0 resection confers enormous benefit for the patient, clinician, and health care system.

TECHNIQUE OF WIDE-FIELD ENDOSCOPIC MUCOSAL RESECTION
Patient and Lesion Positioning

Endoscopic access and lesion orientation should be optimized to maximize procedure success. The working channel of the endoscope is located at the 6-o'clock orientation and, hence, this is the best position for the target tissue. This location also maximizes the effect of the up/down wheel when pushing down for tissue capture. The lesion should also be positioned away from fluid pools, which may require patient position change to supine or right lateral. Retroflexion using a thinner endoscope (pediatric colonoscope or gastroscope) may be necessary to improve access.

Injection Technique

Submucosal injections must be carefully placed to lift the lesion into the lumen and improve access. The first few injections are particularly important because they form the basis for a successful procedure.

- In general, the least accessible area should be targeted first. The lesion should be in the 6-o'clock orientation.
- Position the needle tip tangentially at the interface between the lesion and normal mucosa.
- Ensure the catheter is primed and then ask an assistant to commence injection before entering the mucosa.
- Make a short, swift stab of the mucosa to enter the submucosal plane, which is confirmed by immediate elevation of the mucosa.
- Elevation of the lesion is achieved by gently pulling back on the needle (by pulling on either the injection catheter or colonoscope) and deflecting the tip of the colonoscope up into the lumen while maintaining the needle tip within the submucosal plane.
- We perform 2 to 4 resections for every 1 to 2 sequential injections.
- Submucosal injection outcomes include:
  ○ Successful injection: lesion elevates.
  ○ Intramucosal injection: blue bleb forms without lesion elevation. This is easily torn with the needle tip.

○ Extramural injection: lesion d
○ Intraluminal injection: fluid is
○ Jet sign: a jet of fluid exits the of submucosal fibrosis (SMF).
○ Canyon sign: the lesion remai and the surrounding tissue ele
- An approach to nonlifting lesions
- Excessive injections must be av endoscopic access and limit snar

Resection Technique

Resection needs to be systematic with c tential adverse events such as deep mu incompletely excised polyp (**Figs. 3 and**

- Resect the most inaccessible and c
- Align the snare over the target area, tissue at the edge to reduce the risk
- Push down firmly on the fluid cushio gas. This pressure reduces tension capture.
- Ask an assistant to close the snare s captured tissue, which is fluid filled su ally not possible to transect tissue gre
- We prefer to handle the snare durin invaluable sensory feedback on the sa by 3 maneuvers:
  ○ Relative mobility; the ensnared tissue tive to the adjacent colonic wall.
  ○ Full closure of the snare with a spongy of the surrounding mucosa, deeper tis

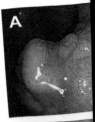
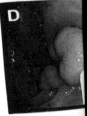

Fig. 3. WF-EMR mucosal injectio ture, (E) expose no evidence of

be co
the sn
○ Fast tr
pulses
A long
SMF,
- Inspect
(discuss

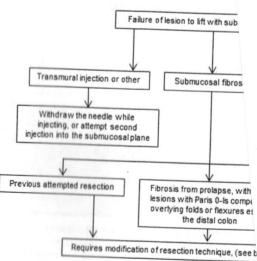

Failure of lesion to lift with sub

Transmural injection or other   Submucosal fibros

Withdraw the needle while injecting, or attempt second injection into the submucosal plane

Previous attempted resection   Fibrosis from prolapse, with lesions with Paris 0-Is comp overlying folds or flexures es the distal colon

Requires modification of resection technique, (see b

Fig. 2. Initial approach to nonlifting lesion following s

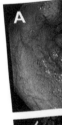

Fig. 4. WF- view of les resection i (F) adjuva

WF-EMR. These processors deliver alternating cycles of high-frequency short-pulse cutting with more prolonged coagulation current and adjust power output according to the impedance signals received from the return electrode. Consequently, the risk of unnecessary deep tissue injury is limited. The energy delivery is optimized to achieve excision of the mucosal neoplasm.

LESION ASSESSMENT

Careful assessment of the lesion before resection is vital because it informs the risk of SMI, submucosal scarring, and endoscopic accessibility. These aspects may mandate an alternate management approach. Suspected superficial SMI may be suitable for endoscopic resection but this should be en bloc, so endoscopic submucosal dissection (ESD) may be preferred or surgery may be more appropriate. Predicted deep SMI is best managed by surgery.

Lesion assessment entails overview and focal interrogation components. In overview Paris morphology and surface topography (granular, nongranular, or mixed) stratify the risk of SMI.[11,20,21] For instance, a homogeneous Paris 0-IIa granular lesion has a low risk of SMI at 1% to 2%, whereas a Paris 0-IIa + IIc nongranular lesion has the highest risk of SMI of up to ~70% (**Fig. 1**).

Focal interrogation of areas at risk of SMI is essential. This interrogation may be classified by the mucosal crypt orifices (the pit pattern) according to the Kudo

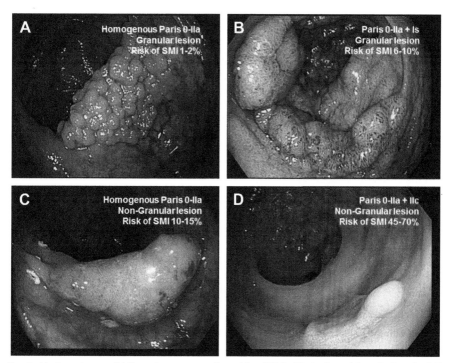

Fig. 1. Various types of LSL and corresponding risk of SMI. (*Data from* Moss A, Bourke MJ, Williams SJ, Hourigan LF, Brown G, Tam W, et al. Endoscopic mucosal resection outcomes and prediction of submucosal cancer from advanced colonic mucosal neoplasia. Gastroenterology 2011;140(7):1909–18; and Uraoka T, Saito Y, Matsuda T, Ikehara H, Gotoda T, Saito D, et al. Endoscopic indications for endoscopic mucosal resection of laterally spreading tumours in the colorectum. Gut 2006;55(11):1592–70.)

classification,[22] the vascular pattern according to the Sano classification,[23] or more recently the Narrow-Band Imaging International Colorectal Endoscopic (NICE) classi-fication.[24] These classification criteria can be used to predict histology and SMI.[11,24,25] Pit pattern types III and IV indicate benign adenoma, whereas pit pattern type V is associated with SMI.

A useful general principle is that a benign lesion has a homogeneous surface pit pattern without any obvious transition line or demarcation zone. SMI may be consid-ered as overt or covert based on endoscopic imaging. A recent advance in lesion assessment is risk stratification for covert SMI; that is, the realization that certain gross LSL morphologies may be stratified for submucosal invasive cancer in the absence of highly suggestive surface endoscopic features, such as type V pit pattern. In a pro-spective study, the following features were associated with increased risk for covert malignancy: distal colon (rectosigmoid location), combined Paris classification (eg, 0-IIa + Is), nongranular surface topography, and increasing lesion size.[26] These new findings can be used to further rationalize which patients undergo EMR or ESD based on local expertise and resources, which is especially pertinent in the rectum, where endoscopic cure of low-risk submucosal cancer by en bloc R0 resection confers enor-mous benefit for the patient, clinician, and health care system.

TECHNIQUE OF WIDE-FIELD ENDOSCOPIC MUCOSAL RESECTION
Patient and Lesion Positioning

Endoscopic access and lesion orientation should be optimized to maximize procedure success. The working channel of the endoscope is located at the 6-o'clock orientation and, hence, this is the best position for the target tissue. This location also maximizes the effect of the up/down wheel when pushing down for tissue capture. The lesion should also be positioned away from fluid pools, which may require patient position change to supine or right lateral. Retroflexion using a thinner endoscope (pediatric co-lonoscope or gastroscope) may be necessary to improve access.

Injection Technique

Submucosal injections must be carefully placed to lift the lesion into the lumen and improve access. The first few injections are particularly important because they form the basis for a successful procedure.

- In general, the least accessible area should be targeted first. The lesion should be in the 6-o'clock orientation.
- Position the needle tip tangentially at the interface between the lesion and normal mucosa.
- Ensure the catheter is primed and then ask an assistant to commence injection before entering the mucosa.
- Make a short, swift stab of the mucosa to enter the submucosal plane, which is confirmed by immediate elevation of the mucosa.
- Elevation of the lesion is achieved by gently pulling back on the needle (by pulling on either the injection catheter or colonoscope) and deflecting the tip of the co-lonoscope up into the lumen while maintaining the needle tip within the submu-cosal plane.
- We perform 2 to 4 resections for every 1 to 2 sequential injections.
- Submucosal injection outcomes include:
  - Successful injection: lesion elevates.
  - Intramucosal injection: blue bleb forms without lesion elevation. This is easily torn with the needle tip.

- ○ Extramural injection: lesion does not elevate despite ongoing injection.
- ○ Intraluminal injection: fluid is seen to escape.
- ○ Jet sign: a jet of fluid exits the lesion at high pressure because of the presence of submucosal fibrosis (SMF).
- ○ Canyon sign: the lesion remains anchored because of the presence of SMF and the surrounding tissue elevates.
- An approach to nonlifting lesions is summarized in **Fig. 2**.
- Excessive injections must be avoided because they can potentially obstruct endoscopic access and limit snare capture.

Resection Technique

Resection needs to be systematic with careful attention at every stage to minimize potential adverse events such as deep mural injury (DMI; discussed later) and islands of incompletely excised polyp (**Figs. 3 and 4** for examples of WF-EMR).

- Resect the most inaccessible and difficult area first.
- Align the snare over the target area, including a 2-mm to 3-mm margin of normal tissue at the edge to reduce the risk of residual tissue.
- Push down firmly on the fluid cushion with the up/down wheel while aspirating gas. This pressure reduces tension on the colonic wall and maximizes tissue capture.
- Ask an assistant to close the snare slowly until resistance is encountered. The captured tissue, which is fluid filled submucosa, should feel spongy. It is generally not possible to transect tissue greater than 10 mm without diathermy.
- We prefer to handle the snare during the final resection because it provides invaluable sensory feedback on the safety of the resection, and this is gauged by 3 maneuvers:
  - ○ Relative mobility; the ensnared tissue should move back and forth freely relative to the adjacent colonic wall.
  - ○ Full closure of the snare with a spongy feel. If it feels hard or there is puckering of the surrounding mucosa, deeper tissue may be captured. This problem can

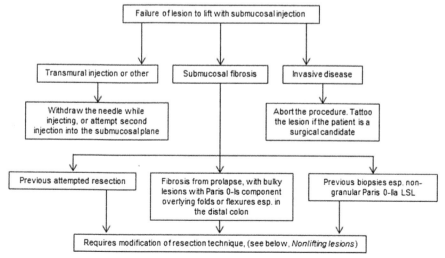

Fig. 2. Initial approach to nonlifting lesion following submucosal injection.

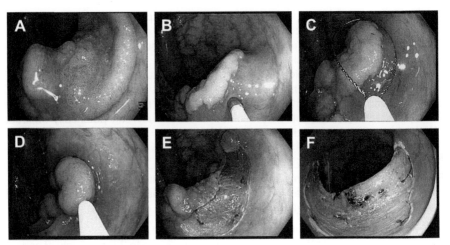

Fig. 3. WF-EMR of a 40-mm Paris 0-IIa granular lesion. (*A*) Lesion overview, (*B*) dynamic submucosal injection, (*C*) snare placement including 2 to 3 mm of normal mucosa, (*D*) tissue capture, (*E*) exposed submucosal tissue following resection, (*F*) completed tissue resection with no evidence of DMI.

be corrected by lifting the captured tissue into the lumen and slightly opening the snare to release the deeper tissue and then closing again.
  ○ Fast transection of the ensnared tissue, which is usually achieved with 1 to 3 pulses of a microprocessor-controlled generator using fractionated current. A longer transection phase raises concern for muscularis propria entrapment, SMF, or invasive disease.
  • Inspect the mucosal defect after every resection for adequacy of resection, DMI (discussed later), and for residual polyp. Irrigating into the defect (with either

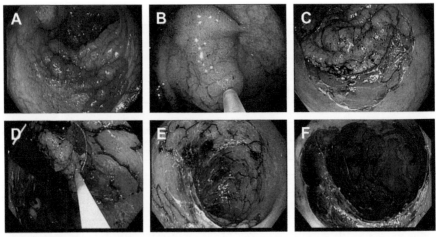

Fig. 4. WF-EMR of 100-mm focally circumferential Paris 0-IIa + Is granular lesion. (*A*) Overview of lesion, (*B*) dynamic submucosal injection, (*C*) exposed submucosal tissue, (*D*) snare resection in retroflexed position, (*E*) completed tissue resection with no evidence of DMI, (*F*) adjuvant thermal ablation to the resection margin (discussed later).

normal saline or the injection solution) expands the defect and may aid in the assessment.

- Use the edge of the mucosal defect as the base for subsequent resection, repeating the steps above until the entire lesion is resected.

INSPECTION OF THE POST–ENDOSCOPIC MUCOSAL RESECTION DEFECT
Deep Mural Injury

DMI, and in particular perforation, is the most serious and feared adverse event of WF-EMR. Perforation or significant DMI occurs in 0.2% to 2.0% of EMR cases[27,28] and is associated with transverse colon location, en bloc resection of lesions greater than or equal to 25 mm, and high-grade dysplasia or submucosal invasive cancer.[28]

The Sydney Classification of DMI[28] (**Fig. 5**, **Table 1**) is a helpful guide for early recognition and management of injury to muscularis propria:

- Carefully inspect the mucosal defect after each resection.
- A normal postresection defect has a homogeneous blue-mat appearance. Herniated or flat nonbleeding blood vessels may be seen.
- Nonstaining areas may be caused by SMF or injury to the muscularis propria and can be evaluated using topical submucosal chromoendoscopy.[29] Gently place the submucosal injection catheter (with the needle withdrawn) against the mucosal defect and irrigate with dye. The dye is taken up by the submucosa and not the muscularis propria. A poorly staining area may define a site of muscle injury and clip closure is advocated to prevent delayed perforation.

Adjuvant Thermal Ablation of the Resection Margin

Thermal ablation of the post-EMR defect margin using snare-tip soft coagulation (STSC) has recently been shown in a prospective multicentre randomized control trial to result in an almost 4-fold reduction in recurrent adenoma (21% vs 6%; *P*<.001) at

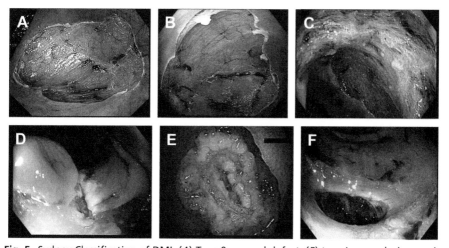

Fig. 5. Sydney Classification of DMI. (*A*) Type 0, normal defect; (*B*) type I, muscularis propria visible but not injured; (*C*) type II, loss of submucosal plane, raising concern for injury to muscularis propria; (*D*) type III, muscularis propria injury with specimen target sign and (*E*) corresponding defect target; (*F*) type IV, hole within white cautery ring, no observed contamination. When contamination is observed it is classified as type V injury.

Table 1
Sydney classification of deep mural injury following wide-field endoscopic mucosal resection and the recommended intervention

DMI Type	Definition	Intervention
Type 0	Normal defect. Blue-mat appearance of obliquely oriented intersecting submucosal connective tissue fibers	No intervention
Type I	Muscularis propria visible, but no mechanical injury	No intervention
Type II	Focal loss of the submucosal plane raising concern for muscularis propria injury or rendering the muscularis propria defect uninterpretable	Clip closure. Patient may be discharged on the same day if there are no signs or symptoms of peritoneal irritation
Type III	Muscularis propria injured, specimen target or defect target identified	
Type IV	Hole within a white cautery ring, no observed contamination	Clip closure. Admission for overnight monitoring should be considered in addition to antibiotics $\pm$ gut rest
Type V	Hole within a white cautery ring, observed contamination	

Adapted from Burgess NG, Bassan MS, McLeod D, Williams SJ, Byth K, Bourke MJ. Deep mural injury and perforation after colonic endoscopic mucosal resection: a new classification and analysis of risk factors. Gut. Oct 2017;66(10):1779–89; with permission.

first surveillance colonoscopy at 6 months.[30] No adverse events were reported. All visible adenoma must be excised before this adjuvant therapy is applied.

Thermal ablation using STSC on completion of EMR is simple to learn and can be completed within a few minutes (**Fig. 6**).

- Expose 1 to 2 mm of the snare tip beyond the snare sheath.
- Align the snare tip tangentially along the resection defect and move gently along the margin applying STSC (soft coagulation mode, effect 4, 80 W, VIO 300D generator; ERBE Elektromedizin) to achieve a homogeneous whitening or denaturation of the mucosa.
- Proceed along the margin with the tip of the colonoscope until the entire margin has been ablated. An aggressive approach may be taken in the rectum, whereas caution is advisable in the proximal colon.

Specimen Retrieval

All specimens should be retrieved for histologic assessment. If there are areas suspicious for SMI, we generally isolate them during resection and place them in a separate specimen jar.

SPECIAL CONSIDERATIONS
Nonlifting Lesions

Lesions with extensive SMF, whether from previous EMR attempts or naive nonlifting lesions (nongranular 0-IIa LSL), can be difficult to excise. Both hot and cold avulsion techniques have been shown to be safe and effective in this scenario,[31,32] with recurrence rates similar to those of lifting lesions. Cold-forceps avulsion and adjuvant STSC (CAST) is performed as follows:

- Isolate the nonlifting area by submucosal injection and snare excision of the surrounding adenomatous and/or normal tissue (**Fig. 7A**).

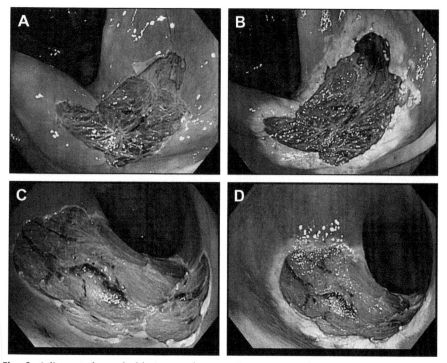

Fig. 6. Adjuvant thermal ablation to the resection margin. After completion of WF-EMR *(A & C)*, the mucosal defect is treated with STSC *(B & D)* (ERBE effect 4, 80 W, VIO 300D generator; ERBE Elektromedizin) to reduce the risk of recurrent adenoma.

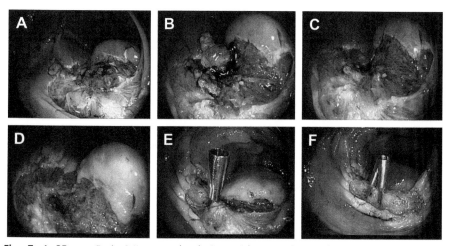

Fig. 7. A 25-mm Paris 0-IIa granular lesion with central SMF from previous resection attempt. The nonlifting area is isolated *(A)*, followed by systematic CAST *(B, C)* until all visible adenoma is excised *(D)*. Two clips deployed over area with DMI (type II) *(E, F)*.

- Systematic cold-forceps avulsion is performed to remove all visible nonlifting adenoma (**Fig. 7**B, C).
- The avulsed area and the margins are then treated with controlled thermal ablation using STSC (ERBE effect 4, 80 W, VIO 300D generator; ERBE Elektromedizin) (**Fig. 7**D).
- The avulsed and coagulated defect is graded according to the Sydney Classification of DMI (discussed earlier). We routinely deploy endoscopic clips over areas with DMI type II and greater. In a prospective study of 100 CAST cases, there were no delayed perforations.[31]

Hot avulsion differs by using hot forceps with electrocautery (Endocut I, 3-1-3 setting; ERBE, Erlangen, Germany) to perform avulsion.[32] Using this technique, no follow-up thermal treatment of the ablation bed is necessary.

Two-Stage Wide-Field Endoscopic Mucosal Resection

Single-session WF-EMR is preferable and is achievable in greater than 95% of cases.[12] It is generally preferred to remove the LSL in a single attempt. Failure of single-session EMR may be caused by SMF, difficult locations, difficult position such as ileocecal valve, and/or anesthetic issues.[12,33,34] Unsuspected covert cancer may also lead to suspension of the resection. If subsequent histology is benign, a follow-up for completion may be performed at 6 to 8 weeks.

Two-stage WF-EMR, whether deliberate or as a salvage therapy following a failed single session, has been shown to be safe and effective.[35] Technical success can be achieved in approximately 85% of cases. SMF is the main challenge. The submucosal plane should be entered away from any area of SMF and then the resection proceeds to the scarred area. Avulsion techniques are necessary in approximately 20% of cases. Complications rates are comparable with those of single-session procedures.

Lesions at the Anorectal Junction

The anorectal junction (ARJ) has somatic sensory innervation and unique venolymphatic drainage directly into the systemic circulation, thus technical adaptations are necessary.[36] These adaptations include:

- Use of a long-acting local anesthetic (eg, ropivacaine 0.5%) within the submucosal injectate to provide anesthesia for 4 hours and provide analgesia for 24 hours. Cardiac monitoring is recommended.
- Prophylactic antibiotics should be used when EMR is performed within 5 cm of the ARJ because of the risk of systemic bacteraemia.[36]
- Submucosal injection followed by tissue resection begins at the ARJ and proceeds proximally. Hemorrhoidal vessels are generally excluded from the ensnared tissue. They are thick walled and tend to be resistant to snare capture.
- Patient position change is helpful to optimize endoscopic access and clear fluid pools. A distal transparent cap may be helpful to optimize lesion exposure in the anal canal.
- Oral analgesia (eg, acetaminophen 1 g every 6 hours) is effective and may be required for a few days. Stool softeners (eg, docusate) should for used for 2 weeks.

Ileocecal Valve Lesions

Access to ileocecal valve (ICV) lesions may be challenging. A retroflexed approach to the ICV (using a pediatric colonoscope or gastroscope, possibly with a distal cap) is necessary for any significant lesion, especially those involving the inferior lip. The terminal ileum must be intubated to delineate the transition zone between adenoma and the villiform ileal tissue. Submucosal injection may facilitate delineation of this transition zone, which may be challenging. Resection starts at the proximal ileal margin. Overinjection should be avoided. Overall technical success is 94%; factors associated with technical failure are ileal infiltration and involvement of both ICV lips.[33] Recurrence is 4-fold,[12,33] so careful and expert follow-up is mandatory.

Periappendiceal Lesions

Lesions involving the appendiceal orifice can be challenging to resect because of the presence of SMF and limited visualization of the proximal/or intra-appendiceal component.[34] Ten-millimeter snares are preferred. Submucosal injection needs to be precise to prevent transmural injection. EMR is generally achievable if the lesion involves less than 50% of the appendiceal orifice and the proximal margin can be visualized.[34] Surgery should be considered for lesions that do not meet these criteria because high-grade dysplasia or cancer may be concealed in the appendix.[34]

Circumferential Lesions

Circumferential colonic lesions are uncommon ($\sim$1%), usually found in the distal colon, and have traditionally been managed surgically. EMR has been proved to be safe and effective[37] using the simple principles described earlier. Post-EMR stricture occurs in up to 50% of cases, particularly if there is preexisting luminal narrowing, such as diverticular disease. Patients are treated with steroid enemas (20 mg of prednisolone sodium phosphate) twice daily for 8 weeks after resection to mitigate stricture formation. Gentle serial balloon dilatation is preferred, beginning with a 10-mm to 12-mm balloon at 2 to 3 weeks after resection. The treatment intervals thereafter are tailored to symptoms and endoscopic response. Serial dilatations are discontinued once a diameter of 15 mm is achieved and maintained.

POSTPROCEDURE CARE

WF-EMR is ideally performed in the morning to allow for several hours of patient monitoring after the procedure, before patient discharge to home.

ADVERSE EVENTS OF WIDE-FIELD ENDOSCOPIC MUCOSAL RESECTION

WF-EMR is associated with several potential adverse events, which are covered more extensively elsewhere in this issue. Adverse events include:

- Perforation: the most serious complication. As a result of technical improvements, knowledge of risk factors, and early recognition, its frequency has declined substantially and should now be less than 1%.[28]
- Intraprocedural bleeding: occurs in approximately 10% of cases and is controlled endoscopically in virtually all cases[26,38] (**Fig 8**).
- Postprocedural bleeding: occurs in 6% to 7% of cases, and resolves spontaneously without colonoscopy in more than 50% cases.[39–42]
- Postprocedural pain is common. Causes include gaseous distension, particularly with use of air; excessive transmural fluid injection; serositis; and perforation.[10,43]

Early recognition and prompt management are essential to mitigate adverse events. Multidisciplinary management, including radiological and surgical consultation, is essential.

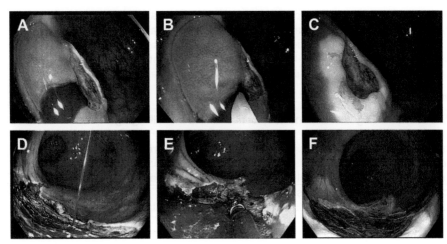

Fig. 8. Minor intraprocedural bleeding (*A*) controlled with STSC (*B*, *C*). Brisk arterial bleeding (*D*) controlled with coagulating forceps grasper (*E*, *F*).

HOW TO PERFORM FOLLOW-UP EXAMINATIONS AFTER WIDE-FIELD ENDOSCOPIC MUCOSAL RESECTION
Residual/Recurrent Adenoma Following Wide-Field Endoscopic Mucosal Resection

Endoscopic surveillance is a critical component of all endoscopic tissue resection techniques. Following WF-EMR, surveillance colonoscopy is usually undertaken at 6 months to carefully assess the scar for any residual/recurrent adenoma (RRA).[44,45] In the largest prospective multicentre study, RRA was observed in 16% of cases at 4 months and 4% at 16 months following EMR.[12] The advent of thermal ablation of the postresection EMR margin has reduced the recurrence to the order of 2% to 5%.[30]

RRA is usually unifocal, diminutive, does not harbor advanced disease, and is readily treated endoscopically.[12] This treatment is usually achieved by snare excision and/or CAST (**Fig. 9**). Risk factors for RRA include lesion size

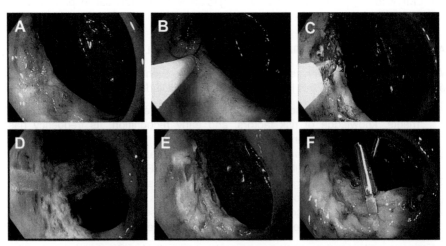

Fig. 9. A 20-mm Paris 0-IIa granular RRA with SMF (*A*). All visible RRA excised by a combination of snare excision and cold avulsion (*B–D*). Resection margin treated with thermal therapy (*E*). Two clips deployed over area with DMI (type II) (*F*).

greater than 40 mm, intraprocedural bleeding, and presence of high-grade dysplasia.[12,46]

Residual/Recurrent Adenoma Is Predictable: The Sydney Endoscopic Mucosal Resection Recurrence Tool

Although current guidelines recommend first follow-up colonoscopy at 4 to 6 months,[47,48] this period can safely be extended for low-risk lesions using the Sydney EMR Recurrence Tool (SERT).[46]

Using prospective, multicentre data, 3 factors (lesion >40 mm, intraprocedural bleeding, and high-grade dysplasia) were identified as independent EMR predictors of endoscopically determined recurrence and were allocated scores of 2, 1, and 1, respectively, to create SERT.[46] Lesions with a SERT score of 0 proved low risk for RRA at 6 months (9.8%) and with minimal increment at 18 months (11.6%). However, lesions with SERT scores of 1 to 4 proved high risk for RRA at 6 months (23% cumulative incidence) and showed considerable increment at 18 months (36.3%).

Therefore, for low-risk lesions (SERT = 0), the first surveillance colonoscopy may safely be performed at 18 months, which has significant economic benefits in

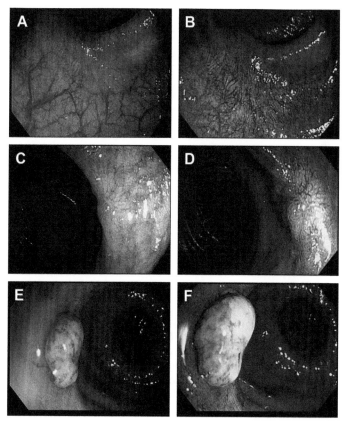

Fig. 10. (*A*) Bland post-EMR scar on white light and (*B*) NBI. (*C, D*) Diminutive RRA on white light and NBI. (*E–H*) Histology-proven inflammatory nodules within post-EMR scar. (*I, J*) Clip artifact on white light and NBI, histology-proven normal mucosa. (*K, L*) Residual clips within post-EMR scar, histology consistent with regenerative mucosa.

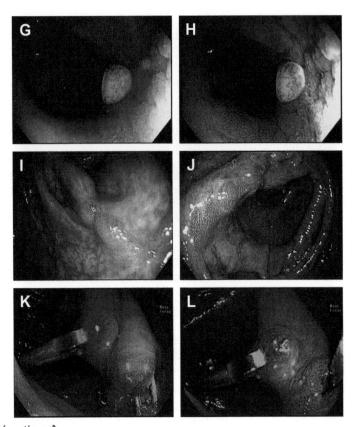

Fig. 10. (*continued*).

addition to the benefits of patient safety and convenience.[46] High-risk lesions (SERT 1–4) should have follow-up surveillance colonoscopies at 6, 18, and 36 months as per current international guidelines.[47,48] These recommendations may change with the advent of thermal ablation of the post-EMR defect margin.

Standardized Endoscopic Mucosal Resection Scar Assessment on Follow-up Examinations

A meticulous standardized assessment of the post-EMR scar using high-definition white light (HD-WL) and narrow band imaging (NBI) can accurately detect RRA with sensitivity, specificity, and negative predictive values of 93.3%, 94.1%, and 98.8%, respectively.[49] This examination includes:

- Identification of the post-EMR scar, typically a pale area with obvious disruption of the regular pit or vascular pattern (**Fig. 10**A, B).
- HD-WL and NBI interrogation of the scar beginning at one edge of the scar and slowly moving across to the other edge.
- Particular attention given to the surface pattern, which should be homogenous. The presence of a transition zone or line may indicate residual adenoma.

Possible findings of post-EMR scar assessment include (**Fig. 10**):

- Bland scar: flat mucosa with normal pit pattern surrounding the scar tissue.
- RRA: adenomatous pit pattern and hypervascular (darker) on NBI with either an elevated or flat morphology.

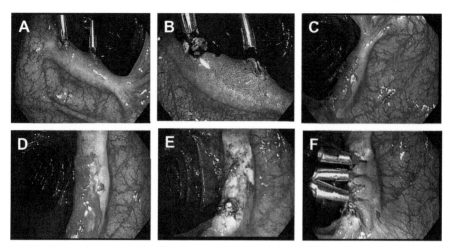

Fig. 11. Clip artifact. (*A, B*) Post-EMR scar with residual clips. (*B*) Pit pattern of nodular mucosa not typical of adenoma. (*C*) Clips removed using a snare, (*D*) nodular mucosa avulsed with cold forceps, (*E*) followed by STSC. (*F*) Three clips deployed over area with DMI (type II). Biopsy specimens were consistent with regenerative mucosa.

- Clip artifact: nodular elevation with a normal pit pattern. This artifact may occur with or without residual clips.[50]
- Inflammatory/regenerative nodules: these can be mistaken for RRA. On close examination there is absence of typical adenomatous pit pattern, and they can be erythematous and friable.
- Inconclusive focal changes.

We generally treat RRA and ambiguous areas such as inflammatory nodules with snare resection and/or CAST (see **Fig. 9**). If residual clips are present, we usually remove them to optimize the assessment of the scar, although this is not mandatory (**Fig. 11**). If the scar is bland on HD-WL and NBI, systematic post-EMR scar biopsies are taken (1 biopsy per 5 mm) to ensure no histologic evidence of RRA. This biopsy step may become unnecessary as further data accumulate.

SUMMARY

WF-EMR is unequivocally the primary management option for noninvasive laterally spreading colorectal lesions. It is safe, highly effective, efficient, and inexpensive when performed by well-trained and experienced endoscopists and their teams. Adjuvant thermal ablation of the post-EMR defect margin significantly reduces adenoma recurrence and should now be considered a standard practice. The risk and timeline of adenoma recurrence can be stratified and surveillance intervals tailored accordingly using the SERT. Recurrent adenoma is accurately detected using a standardized imaging protocol, available to all, and can be effectively treated using simple and safe techniques.

REFERENCES

1. Siegel RL, Fedewa SA, Anderson WF, et al. Colorectal cancer incidence patterns in the United States, 1974-2013. J Natl Cancer Inst 2017;109(8):322–8.
2. Levin B, Lieberman DA, McFarland B, et al. Screening and surveillance for the early detection of colorectal cancer and adenomatous polyps, 2008: a joint

guideline from the American Cancer Society, the US Multi-Society Task Force on Colorectal Cancer, and the American College of Radiology. Gastroenterology 2008;134(5):1570–95.

3. Winawer SJ, Zauber AG, Ho MN, et al. Prevention of colorectal cancer by colonoscopic polypectomy. The National Polyp Study Workgroup. N Engl J Med 1993; 329(27):1977–81.

4. Kahi CJ, Imperiale TF, Juliar BE, et al. Effect of screening colonoscopy on colorectal cancer incidence and mortality. Clin Gastroenterol Hepatol 2009;7(7): 770–5 [quiz 711].

5. Zauber AG, Winawer SJ, O'Brien MJ, et al. Colonoscopic polypectomy and long-term prevention of colorectal-cancer deaths. N Engl J Med 2012;366(8):687–96.

6. Rex DK. Have we defined best colonoscopic polypectomy practice in the United States? Clin Gastroenterol Hepatol 2007;5(6):674–7.

7. Gupta N, Bansal A, Rao D, et al. Prevalence of advanced histological features in diminutive and small colon polyps. Gastrointest Endosc 2012;75(5):1022–30.

8. Repici A, Hassan C, Vitetta E, et al. Safety of cold polypectomy for <10mm polyps at colonoscopy: a prospective multicenter study. Endoscopy 2012;44(1):27–31.

9. Holt BA, Bourke MJ. Wide field endoscopic resection for advanced colonic mucosal neoplasia: current status and future directions. Clin Gastroenterol Hepatol 2012;10(9):969–79.

10. Bourke M. Endoscopic mucosal resection in the colon: a practical guide. Tech Gastrointest Endosc 2011;13:35–49.

11. Moss A, Bourke MJ, Williams SJ, et al. Endoscopic mucosal resection outcomes and prediction of submucosal cancer from advanced colonic mucosal neoplasia. Gastroenterology 2011;140(7):1909–18.

12. Moss A, Williams SJ, Hourigan LF, et al. Long-term adenoma recurrence following wide-field endoscopic mucosal resection (WF-EMR) for advanced colonic mucosal neoplasia is infrequent: results and risk factors in 1000 cases from the Australian Colonic EMR (ACE) study. Gut 2015;64(1):57–65.

13. Klein A, Bourke MJ. Advanced polypectomy and resection techniques. Gastrointest Endosc Clin N A 2015;25(2):303–33.

14. Klein A, Bourke MJ. How to perform high-quality endoscopic mucosal resection during colonoscopy. Gastroenterology 2017;152(3):466–71.

15. Ferlitsch M, Moss A, Hassan C, et al. Colorectal polypectomy and endoscopic mucosal resection (EMR): European Society of Gastrointestinal Endoscopy (ESGE) Clinical Guideline. Endoscopy 2017;49(3):270–97.

16. Ahlenstiel G, Hourigan LF, Brown G, et al. Actual endoscopic versus predicted surgical mortality for treatment of advanced mucosal neoplasia of the colon. Gastrointest Endosc 2014;80(4):668–76.

17. Jayanna M, Burgess NG, Singh R, et al. Cost analysis of endoscopic mucosal resection vs surgery for large laterally spreading colorectal lesions. Clin Gastroenterol Hepatol 2016;14(2):271–8.e1-2.

18. Moss A, Bourke MJ, Metz AJ. A randomized, double-blind trial of succinylated gelatin submucosal injection for endoscopic resection of large sessile polyps of the colon. Am J Gastroenterol 2010;105(11):2375–82.

19. Bahin FF, Rasouli KN, Byth K, et al. Prediction of clinically significant bleeding following wide-field endoscopic resection of large sessile and laterally spreading colorectal lesions: a clinical risk score. Am J Gastroenterol 2016;111(8):1115–22.

20. Uraoka T, Saito Y, Matsuda T, et al. Endoscopic indications for endoscopic mucosal resection of laterally spreading tumours in the colorectum. Gut 2006; 55(11):1592–7.

21. The Paris endoscopic classification of superficial neoplastic lesions: esophagus, stomach, and colon: November 30 to December 1, 2002. Gastrointest Endosc 2003;58(6 Suppl):S3–43.

22. Kudo S, Hirota S, Nakajima T, et al. Colorectal tumours and pit pattern. J Clin Pathol 1994;47(10):880–5.

23. Sano Y, Ikematsu H, Fu KI, et al. Meshed capillary vessels by use of narrow-band imaging for differential diagnosis of small colorectal polyps. Gastrointest Endosc 2009;69(2):278–83.

24. Hayashi N, Tanaka S, Hewett DG, et al. Endoscopic prediction of deep submucosal invasive carcinoma: validation of the narrow-band imaging international colorectal endoscopic (NICE) classification. Gastrointest Endosc 2013;78(4):625–32.

25. Matsuda T, Fujii T, Saito Y, et al. Efficacy of the invasive/non-invasive pattern by magnifying chromoendoscopy to estimate the depth of invasion of early colorectal neoplasms. Am J Gastroenterol 2008;103(11):2700–6.

26. Burgess NG, Hourigan LF, Zanati SA, et al. Risk stratification for covert invasive cancer among patients referred for colonic endoscopic mucosal resection: a large multicenter cohort. Gastroenterology 2017;153(3):732–42.e1.

27. Raju GS, Saito Y, Matsuda T, et al. Endoscopic management of colonoscopic perforations (with videos). Gastrointest Endosc 2011;74(6):1380–8.

28. Burgess NG, Bassan MS, McLeod D, et al. Deep mural injury and perforation after colonic endoscopic mucosal resection: a new classification and analysis of risk factors. Gut 2017;66(10):1779–89.

29. Holt BA, Jayasekeran V, Sonson R, et al. Topical submucosal chromoendoscopy defines the level of resection in colonic EMR and may improve procedural safety (with video). Gastrointest Endosc 2013;77(6):949–53.

30. Klein A, Tate DJ, Jayasekeran V, et al. Thermal ablation of mucosal defect margins reduces adenoma recurrence after colonic endoscopic mucosal resection. Gastroenterology 2018. https://doi.org/10.1053/j.gastro.2018.10.003.

31. Tate DJ, Bahin FF, Desomer L, et al. Cold-forceps avulsion with adjuvant snare-tip soft coagulation (CAST) is an effective and safe strategy for the management of non-lifting large laterally spreading colonic lesions. Endoscopy 2018;50(1):52–62.

32. Kumar V, Broadley H, Rex DK. Safety and efficacy of hot avulsion as an adjunct to endoscopic mucosal resection (with videos). Gastrointest Endosc 2018. https://doi.org/10.1016/j.gie.2018.11.032.

33. Nanda KS, Tutticci N, Burgess NG, et al. Endoscopic mucosal resection of laterally spreading lesions involving the ileocecal valve: technique, risk factors for failure, and outcomes. Endoscopy 2015;47(8):710–8.

34. Tate DJ, Desomer L, Awadie H, et al. EMR of laterally spreading lesions around or involving the appendiceal orifice: technique, risk factors for failure, and outcomes of a tertiary referral cohort (with video). Gastrointest Endosc 2018;87(5):1279–88.e2.

35. Tate DJ, Desomer L, Hourigan LF, et al. Two-stage endoscopic mucosal resection is a safe and effective salvage therapy after a failed single-session approach. Endoscopy 2017;49(9):888–98.

36. Holt BA, Bassan MS, Sexton A, et al. Advanced mucosal neoplasia of the anorectal junction: endoscopic resection technique and outcomes (with videos). Gastrointest Endosc 2014;79(1):119–26.

37. Tutticci N, Klein A, Sonson R, et al. Endoscopic resection of subtotal or completely circumferential laterally spreading colonic adenomas: technique, caveats, and outcomes. Endoscopy 2016;48(5):465–71.

38. Fahrtash-Bahin F, Holt BA, Jayasekeran V, et al. Snare tip soft coagulation achieves effective and safe endoscopic hemostasis during wide-field endoscopic resection of large colonic lesions (with videos). Gastrointest Endosc 2013;78(1):158–63.e1.

39. Bahin FF, Naidoo M, Williams SJ, et al. Prophylactic endoscopic coagulation to prevent bleeding after wide-field endoscopic mucosal resection of large sessile colon polyps. Clin Gastroenterol Hepatol 2015;13(4):724–30.e1-2.

40. Burgess NG, Metz AJ, Williams SJ, et al. Risk factors for intraprocedural and clinically significant delayed bleeding after wide-field endoscopic mucosal resection of large colonic lesions. Clin Gastroenterol Hepatol 2014;12(4):651–61.e1-3.

41. Burgess NG, Williams SJ, Hourigan LF, et al. A management algorithm based on delayed bleeding after wide-field endoscopic mucosal resection of large colonic lesions. Clin Gastroenterol Hepatol 2014;12(9):1525–33.

42. Metz AJ, Bourke MJ, Moss A, et al. Factors that predict bleeding following endoscopic mucosal resection of large colonic lesions. Endoscopy 2011;43(6):506–11.

43. Bassan MS, Holt B, Moss A, et al. Carbon dioxide insufflation reduces number of postprocedure admissions after endoscopic resection of large colonic lesions: a prospective cohort study. Gastrointest Endosc 2013;77(1):90–5.

44. Pohl H, Srivastava A, Bensen SP, et al. Incomplete polyp resection during colonoscopy-results of the complete adenoma resection (CARE) study. Gastroenterology 2013;144(1):74–80.e1.

45. Robertson DJ, Lieberman DA, Winawer SJ, et al. Colorectal cancers soon after colonoscopy: a pooled multicohort analysis. Gut 2014;63(6):949–56.

46. Tate DJ, Desomer L, Klein A, et al. Adenoma recurrence after piecemeal colonic EMR is predictable: the Sydney EMR recurrence tool. Gastrointest Endosc 2017; 85(3):647–56.e6.

47. Hassan C, Quintero E, Dumonceau JM, et al. Post-polypectomy colonoscopy surveillance: European Society of Gastrointestinal Endoscopy (ESGE) guideline. Endoscopy 2013;45(10):842–51.

48. Lieberman DA, Rex DK, Winawer SJ, et al. Guidelines for colonoscopy surveillance after screening and polypectomy: a consensus update by the US Multi-Society Task Force on Colorectal Cancer. Gastroenterology 2012;143(3):844–57.

49. Desomer L, Tutticci N, Tate DJ, et al. A standardized imaging protocol is accurate in detecting recurrence after EMR. Gastrointest Endosc 2017;85(3):518–26.

50. Pellise M, Desomer L, Burgess NG, et al. The influence of clips on scars after EMR: clip artifact. Gastrointest Endosc 2016;83(3):608–16.

How to Learn and Perform Endoscopic Submucosal Dissection and Full-Thickness Resection in the Colorectum in the United States

Kavel Visrodia, MD, Amrita Sethi, MD*

KEYWORDS

- Endoscopic submucosal dissection • Rectum • Training • Cancer • Dysplasia
- Pathology • United States

KEY POINTS

- Endoscopic submucosal dissection (ESD) is a well-established technique originally developed in Japan to treat early gastric cancer that has now been applied throughout the gastrointestinal tract, including the colorectum.
- The Western endoscopist must face unique barriers in the path to learning ESD and incorporating it into practice, but should not be discouraged because it is still possible with commitment and use of increasingly available resources.
- ESD begins with the appropriate selection of cases that are most likely to harbor superficially invasive cancer, and benefit from ESD over endoscopic mucosal resection or surgery.
- Learning and performing ESD in the colorectum will continue to be facilitated by the ongoing development of techniques, accessories, and devices specific for this purpose.
- The recent introduction of a device for full-thickness resection provides an alternative to treating lesions not amenable to standard endoscopic mucosal resection or ESD.

INTRODUCTION

Colonoscopy and endoscopic resection have reduced the incidence and mortality related to colorectal cancer. Endoscopic resection has evolved from simple polypectomy to endoscopic mucosal resection (EMR). However, large colonic lesions that may harbor superficial cancer or fibrosis are not amenable to en bloc removal by

Disclosure: A. Sethi is a consultant for Boston Scientific and Olympus. K. Visrodia has no disclosures.
Division of Digestive and Liver Disease, Columbia University Medical Center – New York Presbyterian Hospital, 630 West 168th Street, Box 83, P&S3-401, New York, NY 10032, USA
* Corresponding author.
E-mail address: As3614@columbia.edu

snare-based methods. Endoscopic submucosal dissection (ESD) is a technique pioneered in Japan for the resection of gastric cancer to address the limitations of EMR. ESD is not restricted by size and allows precise histopathologic assessment of resection margins. Moreover, ESD is associated with a low rate of tumor recurrence with the potential for curative resection, effectively reducing the number of additional procedures and even surgery.[1] ESD has now been applied throughout the gastrointestinal tract, including the colorectum. Although ESD is now a well-established technique among endoscopists in Eastern countries, it remains technically challenging and over the last decade has been slow to gain traction in the West. There are several unique barriers that Western endoscopists must navigate in their path to learning ESD, but these should not deter those interested in learning ESD.

Techniques in ESD, particularly in the colorectum, have also evolved as experience blossoms. These variations in techniques have particularly developed to manage larger and more complex lesions in the colorectum. In addition, full-thickness resection has emerged as a method to handle colorectal resections that cannot be completed by standard ESD techniques because of scarring or potentially deeper invasion. This article reviews challenges and methods to learning ESD in the United States, and provides a primer on performing ESD and full-thickness resection in the colorectum for the avid endoscopist.

TRAINING

Unlike our colleagues in the East, there are several challenges Western endoscopists may face while attempting to learn ESD or incorporate it into practice. Some of these barriers are inherent to regional variations in disease patterns, particularly the relatively low incidence of early gastric cancers in the West. Although Western countries have a higher incidence of colorectal lesions, these are often technically more challenging and, therefore, less than ideal for those beginning to learn ESD. Other challenges include the significant time commitment to learn and incorporate these much lengthier procedures into practice, more limited access to ESD experts and training centers, acceptance by multidisciplinary team members (eg, Oncology, Surgery) and the institution, lack of guidance in the United States as to indications for ESD, lack of reimbursement codes, and more limited availability of ESD devices (eg, knives) because of regulations. Nonetheless, endoscopists should not be dismayed as significant progress is being made in many of these areas and it is still possible to learn and practice ESD in the United States.

Prerequisites to Learning Endoscopic Submucosal Dissection

Before attempting to learn ESD it is essential to have a thorough understanding of EMR, as many principles of resection and scope control still apply. Competency in management of adverse events such as perforation and bleeding is also mandatory, although more advanced methods can be acquired during ESD training itself. Though not currently considered a prerequisite but rather a component of ESD training, proficiency in lesion identification and classification is highly beneficial in ensuring proper patient selection. Fundamentals in electrocautery and electrosurgery are also useful tools with which to enter into ESD training.

Training Models for Endoscopic Submucosal Dissection

There is no standardized approach to learning ESD, although Japanese training centers have adopted a Master-Apprentice model.[2] This is a step-up approach taken by fellows dedicated to learning ESD, and typically requires several years (and high volumes of patients) before proficiency in ESD is achieved. It begins with a cognitive period of learning ESD principles (indications, limitations, technique, and adverse events), followed by an observership with a master performing a substantial number of ESD cases. The learner then begins assisting an expert during cases to familiarize him or herself further with technique and the use of equipment including knives, submucosal injectants, and electrosurgical units and settings. At some institutions, this may be followed by supervised ESD cases in ex vivo and live animal models. Finally, the learner begins performing ESD in humans, with close supervision and working in tandem with the expert throughout the case. Cases are selected based on technical ease, starting with gastric lesions (preferably in the distal stomach). A minimum of 20 to 30 cases is typically recommended before independent practice or attempting colorectal cases.[3–6]

In the United States a Master-Apprentice model is not feasible, as dedicated ESD fellowships do not currently exist. Nonetheless, a common pathway for learning ESD has emerged with a sort of "stepwise" approach different from that of Eastern counterparts.[2] Much of the initial ESD theory can be achieved through lectures, live courses, self-learning by studying review articles, ESD textbooks (available in English[7]), and online videos. As with other endoscopic techniques, endoscopy courses aimed at teaching ESD are becoming increasingly available, through gastrointestinal (GI) societies such as the American Society for Gastrointestinal Endoscopy and the American College of Gastroenterology, as well as courses offered by individual institutions or industry. These courses are staffed by ESD experts who may perform live cases or review videos, which somewhat offers an observership experience. Additional course systems have been established that not only suggest attendance at multiple sequential courses but also provide a guide to hands-on experience that moves from an ex vivo model to a live animal model, and finally to proctored cases. However, a condensed period of observing an expert performing several ESD cases, whether at a high-volume center in Japan or more locally, is still likely to be beneficial.[8] Hands-on workshops are often integrated with these courses, and also are available at major scientific conferences, offering a chance to develop skills under expert guidance. If real-time supervision by an ESD expert is not possible, sending recordings for feedback at a later time can be helpful but requires significant mentor commitment.[9]

A wide range of models for ESD training exist from ex vivo models, such as those established by Endosim (www.endosim.com), to live animal models. Access to an animal laboratory is likely a critical component for United States endoscopists to practice and refine their ESD technique. Several artificial tissue and ex vivo models exist, but opportunities to practice on live animals that better simulate peristalsis, bleeding, and respiratory movement should be sought. Training specific to the colorectum, however, remains challenging because live animal models such as porcine models do not provide adequate simulation of human colorectal tissue. Bovine specimens have been alternatively used for the colorectum, particularly when training to use innovation such as the Full-Thickness Resection Device (FTRD; OVESCO Endoscopy, Tübingen, Germany) and other new resection platforms.

Innovative work is currently being performed in the area of skills simulation. For example, data regarding use of the TEST (Thompson Endoscopic Skills Trainer) box demonstrates a strong correlation between higher TEST performance skills and higher levels of gastric ESD skills as defined by higher procedure time/lesion size and lower complication rates, suggesting that such a model can be used to facilitate improved ESD skills.[10] Virtual reality simulators using haptic technology are also being developed for training in ESD, where they have been widely used in laparoscopic training programs.[11]

Initial human cases should be proctored by an ESD expert and be carefully selected based on anticipated complexity. Owing to the relative lack of suitable gastric lesions in the West, rectal lesions may be selected in lieu, as ESD of rectal lesions by beginners has been shown to be feasible and safe.[12] As with any endoscopic procedure, the indication for ESD should be clear and include a thorough discussion of the risks and benefits with the patient.

After the first few cases of ESD have been accomplished, it may be beneficial to revisit ESD courses and/or observe live cases by experts to address unanticipated challenges and refine one's skill set. Meanwhile, endoscopists should be cognizant of their procedural outcomes (eg, rates of en bloc, R0 and curative resection rates, adverse events) to ensure appropriate progression of skills and case selection. Unfortunately, no defined competency outcomes have been established in the United States, although some accepted definitions of proficiency include R0 resection rate greater than 80%, dissection speed 9 cm/h, and complication rate less than 10%.[13,14] In addition, studies examining learning curves have been limited to those with a single endoscopist, which limits generalizability. Nonetheless, one study that examined a specific training program in ESD that involved a 12-month training period in which time 5 observational and supervised studies as well as 24 animal procedures were done, demonstrated excellent competency outcomes, particularly in rectal lesions as defined by outcome measures already listed.[15]

As the endoscopist builds proficiency in ESD, he or she can decide to gradually accept more technically challenging cases. These may be lesions that are larger and/or in less accessible areas of the gut such as the esophagus, gastric cardia/fundus, or upstream colon. Collaboration with both surgeons and pathologists is critical in assisting with proper patient selection as well as ensuring appropriate adjuvant care in the cases of upstaged lesions or adverse events. ESD requires a serious long-term commitment, and to build and sustain one's skill set it is recommended that endoscopists maintain a steady volume of ESD procedures.

INDICATIONS

ESD in the colorectum begins with careful and appropriate selection of cases that stand to benefit the most from ESD over EMR or surgery. These are typically lesions with suspected superficially invasive cancer and low risk of nodal metastases. By definition, these are lesions limited to the superficial-most third of submucosa (SM1) with less than 1000 μm of submucosal invasion. This can be predicted using one of several available classification systems, including Paris, Kudo pit pattern, and Narrow-band Imaging International Colorectal Endoscopic classifications. A thorough discussion of these classification systems can be found elsewhere and are not reviewed at this time. In addition, ongoing debate regarding indications for colorectal ESD is discussed elsewhere and thus is not tackled in this article. Suffice it to say that guidelines in the United States are lacking in comparison with our European and Asian colleagues.

PREPROCEDURAL CONSIDERATIONS AND EQUIPMENT PREPARATION

As with any endoscopic procedure, patients' medical histories should be reviewed and optimized for anesthesia and endoscopy. Ideally, antiplatelet agents should be held but may need to be continued based on a discussion with the referring provider or cardiologist regarding the patient's risk for thromboembolism. Prophylactic antibiotics are not necessary, but should be administered if muscle wall injury is suspected.

Performing ESD in the colorectum follows the same principles as in the upper GI tract, though in general is more challenging because of the thinner colonic wall and associated risk of perforation, folds, and potential for paradoxic movement of the endoscope. A standard upper endoscope may be used for rectal and left-sided lesions, whereas a pediatric colonoscope may be necessary for more proximal lesions. An adult colonoscope may limit retroflexion if required to dissect the proximal edge of a lesion. In a tortuous colon, a balloon-assisted enteroscope may be necessary.

A soft, translucent cap should be fitted to the tip of the endoscope to assist with widening of the submucosal space, tamponading small surrounding vessels, and stabilizing the endoscope tip. Knives of various designs are available, each with desirable properties depending on the lesion, and endoscopist preference and skill (**Fig. 1**). Of note, the Flush knife (Fujifilm, Tokyo, Japan), Hybrid knives (I and T types; ERBE, Marietta, GA, USA), and DualKnife-J (Olympus, Tokyo, Japan) allow simultaneous injection of submucosal fluid without the need to exchange for a needle.

Various solutions for submucosal injection also exist, all more viscous than normal saline and designed to provide a more durable submucosal lift. In the United States, 2 popular solutions include Hespan or Voluven (typically used for volume resuscitation in

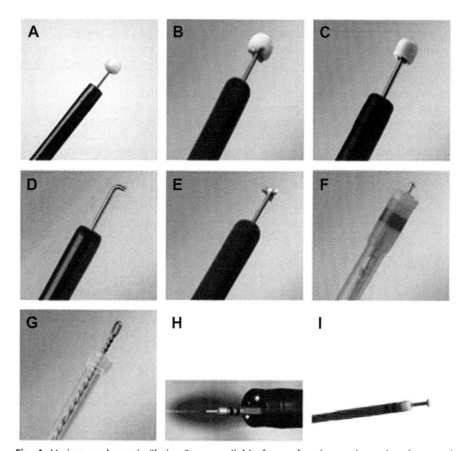

Fig. 1. Various endoscopic "knives" are available for performing endoscopic submucosal dissection. (*A*) ITKnife; (*B*) ITKnife2; (*C*) ITKnife nano; (*D*) HookKnife; (*E*) TTKnife; (*F*) DualKnife; (*G*) FlexKnife; (*H*) HybridKnife I type; (*I*) HybridKnife T type. (*Courtesy of* [*A–G*] Olympus America, Center Valley, PA, with permission; and [*H*, *I*] ©Erbe Elektromedizin GmbH.)

trauma patients) particularly when using jet knives as they are stocked in 500-mL bags. Hyaluronic acid is also commonly used, with a small amount of indigo carmine (or methylene blue) and variably epinephrine added to help visualize the submucosal layer and control bleeding. The electrosurgical unit should be configured for mucosal incision, submucosal dissection, and coagulation settings. Settings tend to vary by endoscopist preference and can be adjusted during the procedure. Hemostatic and closure accessories or devices should be readily available in case of bleeding or perforation. Because of the lengthier procedure time and potential for perforation, carbon dioxide insufflation is considered essential in performing ESD, regardless of location.

TECHNIQUE

As experience with ESD has blossomed and techniques, particularly in the colorectum, have evolved, some basic components remain standard and should be mastered by novice ESD practitioners. Once the lesion is identified, the approach to dissection should be reassessed. The patient should be repositioned and the endoscope should be torqued such that the lesion is positioned to allow the lesion to fall toward the lumen with gravity as resection progresses. Typically the borders are well delineated, and lesion marking is not necessary as taught in the upper GI tract. The initial mucosal incision can be made from either the proximal (oral) or distal (anal) side depending on ease, and the lesion should be lifted accordingly (**Fig. 2**A). Unlike ESD for upper GI lesions, beginning with a fully circumferential incision can result in more consequential leak of submucosal fluid and hinder subsequent submucosal dissection. Therefore, a partial circumferential incision is commonly used to initiate ESD in colorectal lesions. Once a partial mucosal incision is made (at least 5 mm from the edge of the lesion), submucosal dissection follows

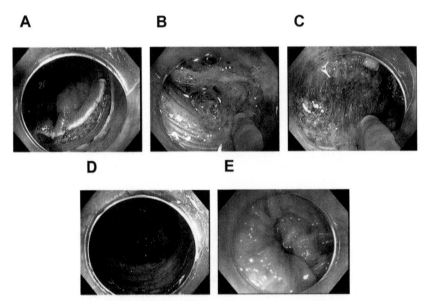

Fig. 2. (*A*) Initial partial circumferential mucosal incision in retroflexion of a 40-mm laterally spreading tumor in the sigmoid colon. (*B, C*) Submucosal dissection. (*D*) Postresection ulcer. (*E*) Follow-up at 1 year without evidence of residual/recurrent polyp.

along the inner edge of the incision until the submucosal space is entered with the cap.

Submucosal dissection is then performed, during which time the lesion should be approached in parallel to the plane of the colonic wall as opposed to perpendicularly and risking perforation (**Fig. 2**B, C). Fine maneuvering of the scope is preferred to moving the knife itself and allows for steady dissection within a consistent plane. Identification of folds is critical in the colorectum, and can often be easier to navigate by remaining close to the muscle wall and dissecting parallel to the muscle layer while taking care not to perforate. It is important to maintain adequate visibility during dissection, periodically reinjecting to expand and visualize the submucosal space. The endoscopist should strive to dissect along the deepest third of submucosa closest to the muscle layer to maximize the depth of resection and potential for R0 resection (**Fig. 2**D, E). Any visible vessels encountered can be prophylactically treated using a cautery effect on the knife or by switching to Coagraspers (Olympus, Tokyo, Japan), because significant bleeding can result in hematoma and obscure the submucosal space. Circumferential incision and submucosal dissection is performed stepwise to complete the resection.

An alternative approach to colorectal ESD, known as the pocket creation method, aims to further reduce submucosal fluid dispersal and improve traction during dissection.[16] This is performed by creating an approximately 20-mm incision that is 10 mm from the distal edge of the lesion following submucosal injection. The submucosal space is entered and submucosal dissection performed through the greater part of the lesion. Additional mucosal incision and submucosal dissection are then used to open the lower edge of the lesion (based on gravity). This is then repeated for the upper edge of the lesion, completing the en bloc resection.

Other Techniques

In an effort to reduce the technical difficulty and procedural duration of ESD, alternative techniques have been described. One of these involves circumferential incision with limited or no submucosal dissection followed by use of a snare to resect the lesion. This approach has been referred to as the hybrid-knife–assisted technique, ESD with snaring, or simplified ESD.[17] This technique may be best suited for medium-sized lesions ranging from 3 to 4 cm or containing fibrosis. Scissor-type devices such as the Clutch Cutter (Fujifilm, Tokyo, Japan) and Stag-Beetle (Sumitomo-Bakelite, Tokyo, Japan) have recently become available; these allow more precise grasping of tissue before cutting and therefore may be more forgiving for novice ESD performers or more suitable for certain situations.

Traction Methods

One significant limitation of ESD in comparison with surgery is the lack of the surgeon's "left hand" that is used to provide traction, which helps improve visibility and facilitates dissection given tension now applied to the tissue. Endoscopic methods to enhance retraction of the lesion to facilitate submucosal dissection, beyond use of the cap, have also been described. One method applies traction by first clipping a rubber band to the margin of the tumor, then using a second clip to attach the end of the rubber band to the opposite colon wall. Similarly, string or dental floss can be attached to the tumor edge, with the endoscopy assistant applying gentle tension on the end to provide traction. Alternatively, a thin transnasal endoscope can be simultaneously inserted and used to provide traction on the clip using a snare. Tissue-retraction systems to assist with retraction have also recently been introduced. These include the ORISE TRS device (Boston Scientific, Marlborough, MA, USA) and

DiLumen (Lumendi, London, UK) systems. Interestingly, technique details vary when using these systems, such as not using a cap for traction as it is provided through dedicated channels and with specified grasping forceps. In addition, the movements used to dissect, given alternative forms of traction, may be different from the basic techniques already described. It is unclear how these new platforms and accessories may alter the manner in which ESD trainees learn their skills and follow their learning curves in comparison with traditional techniques.

POST RESECTION

After ESD is complete, the resection bed should be carefully inspected for any visible vessels and treated accordingly. If cautery is used, "soft" coagulation is recommended to minimize the risk of perforation or postpolypectomy syndrome. Perforations should be closed, typically using the through-the-scope clips, although over-the-scope clips and endoscopic suturing devices may be necessary for larger (>2 cm) perforations. Those training in ESD should have mastery of these closure techniques and for this reason, teaching of various closure methods is often incorporated into hands-on courses.

The specimen should be removed and pinned by the endoscopist to cork or foam to prevent curling and facilitate pathologist evaluation of margins. Depending on the size of the resection and procedural risk factors, it may be reasonable to admit the patient for overnight observation.

FULL-THICKNESS RESECTION IN THE COLORECTUM

Despite best efforts, there are certain colorectal lesions that may not be resectable by ESD methods. Endoscopic full-thickness resection (EFTR) is a method that was realized after experience with closure of NOTES (natural orifice transluminal endoscopic surgery) procedures occurred, whereby complete full-thickness closure was performed. In the United States there is really only one approved dedicated full-thickness device, the FTRD (**Fig. 3**). This device, a modification of the OTSC (Over The Scope Clip; OVESCO) manifests the "close-then-resect" techniques of EFTR, whereby serosal-to-serosal closure is performed first, followed by resection of the tissue above the closed area. The FTRD is currently only indicated in the colorectum in the United States. Accepted indications for EFTR in the colorectum include recurrent adenoma where prior EMR or ESD had been performed, adenoma in which no lift can be achieved with injection signifying either fibrosis or deeper submucosal invasion, superficial colonic malignancy, and submucosal tumors. Owing to the size of the cap of the FTRD, resectable lesions are considered to be those less than 3 cm. Lesions that are larger can be partially resected until they fall within this acceptable range.[18,19]

The FTRD device has several components that require careful and specific assembly. These parts include a 14-mm OTSC clip that is mounted on a 23-mm clear cap. A snare that runs along the outside of the scope is also mounted along the rim of the cap. The device is loaded onto the scope in the same manner as the regular OTSC cap or banding devices and is connected to a deployment wheel that is seated in the biopsy channel. A plastic sleeve is unfurled over the entire length of the scope, thereby covering the snare. The sleeve, and subsequently the snare, is secured along the length of the scope, preventing kinking or looping of the snare as the scope is being advanced through the colon. In addition the packaging contains a marking device that is used before resection to provide visible margins to the lesion as well as grabbers that are used to pull the lesion into the cap.

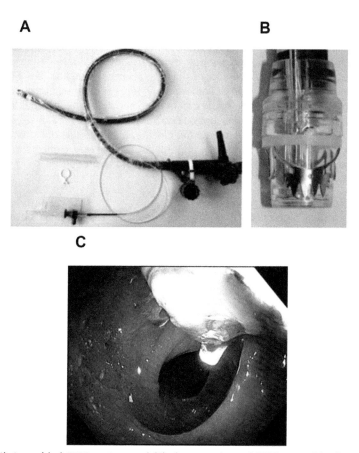

Fig. 3. (*A*) Assembled FTRD system and (*B*) close-up view of FTRD cap with clip and integrated snare. (*C*) Final image following successful deployment of the clip and resection of tissue, with serosal edges visible within the borders of the clip. (*Courtesy of* [*A, B*] FTRD® is a registered trademark of Ovesco Endoscopy AG, a company based in Tubingen, Germany.)

Because of the coordination of the multiple parts of the FTRD, the technique is specific and the company requires dedicated training before using the device. The steps are as follows. First, marking, using the marking device, is made circumferentially around the lesion. This is usually performed through a preresection colonoscope that is advanced to the lesion. It is recommended that a second scope is loaded with the device and kept to the side until the plan for resection is confirmed. When it is decided to proceed with resection, the prepared scope is advanced to the lesion. At this point the grabbers are used to pull the lesion into the cap until the previously made markings are visible and perceived to be within the cap. A coordinated effort involving 3 team members is critical to the next steps. Someone is assigned to hold the grabbers in a closed position. Once it is decided that enough of the lesion is within the cap, the clip is deployed, followed very quickly by closing of the snare and the use of cautery to cut the lesion. Once the lesion has been resected, the grabbers are maintained in a closed position and the scope is withdrawn with the specimen lying just inside the cap. The best way to ensure that the steps are carried out in the correct order and in a coordinated fashion is to assign a different responsibility to an individual team member. All members should undergo training with the device. A "dummy" device that can be used to ensure that apparatus can be advanced to the lesion itself is also available. The resection site should be re-examined to ensure proper deployment. If performed correctly, the serosal edges can be seen within borders of the clip itself, which confirms both closure and successful full-thickness resection (see **Fig. 3**C). In the unfortunate event that the clip did not properly deploy or immediately became dislodged with consequent opening of the defect, care should be taken to put the patient in a position such that fluid or stool contents do not pool into the area. A second OTSC can be deployed if needed to complete the closure, although this does require withdrawal of the scope again to fit the clip apparatus on the scope. Patients undergoing FTRD should receive antibiotics at least at the time of the procedure.

SUMMARY

ESD is a well-established but technically challenging technique that is slowly permeating into Western endoscopy. Inherent limitations make learning difficult but not impossible for the Western endoscopist. For the committed and resourceful endoscopist, ESD can be successfully learned and incorporated into practice. Moreover, improvement in techniques and devices are likely to ease the learning curve while improving procedural duration, safety, and efficacy of colorectal ESD.

REFERENCES

1. Fujiya M, Tanaka K, Dokoshi T, et al. Efficacy and adverse events of EMR and endoscopic submucosal dissection for the treatment of colon neoplasms: a meta-analysis of studies comparing EMR and endoscopic submucosal dissection. Gastrointest Endosc 2015;81:583–95.
2. Kotzev AI, Yang D, Draganov PV. How to master endoscopic submucosal dissection in the USA. Dig Endosc 2019;31:94–100.
3. Kakushima N, Fujishiro M, Kodashima S, et al. A learning curve for endoscopic submucosal dissection of gastric epithelial neoplasms. Endoscopy 2006;38: 991–5.
4. Yamamoto S, Uedo N, Ishihara R, et al. Endoscopic submucosal dissection for early gastric cancer performed by supervised residents: assessment of feasibility and learning curve. Endoscopy 2009;41:923–8.
5. Sakamoto T, Saito Y, Fukunaga S, et al. Learning curve associated with colorectal endoscopic submucosal dissection for endoscopists experienced in gastric endoscopic submucosal dissection. Dis Colon Rectum 2011;54:1307–12.
6. Niimi K, Fujishiro M, Goto O, et al. Safety and efficacy of colorectal endoscopic submucosal dissection by the trainee endoscopists. Dig Endosc 2012; 24(Suppl 1):154–8.
7. Fukami N. Endoscopic submucosal dissection: principles and practice. New York: Springer; 2015.
8. Draganov PV, Chang M, Coman RM, et al. Role of observation of live cases done by Japanese experts in the acquisition of ESD skills by a western endoscopist. World J Gastroenterol 2014;20:4675–80.
9. Bhatt A, Abe S, Kumaravel A, et al. Video-based supervision for training of endoscopic submucosal dissection. Endoscopy 2016;48:711–6.
10. Tamai N, Aihara H, Kato M, et al. Competency assessment for gastric endoscopic submucosal dissection using an endoscopic part-task training box. Surg Endosc 2018. [Epub ahead of print]. https://doi.org/10.1007/s00464-018-6548-7.

11. Cetinsaya B, Gromski MA, Lee S, et al. A task and performance analysis of endoscopic submucosal dissection (ESD) surgery. Surg Endosc 2019;33:592–606.

12. Yang DH, Jeong GH, Song Y, et al. The feasibility of performing colorectal endoscopic submucosal dissection without previous experience in performing gastric endoscopic submucosal dissection. Dig Dis Sci 2015;60:3431–41.

13. Hotta K, Oyama T, Akamatsu T, et al. A comparison of outcomes of endoscopic submucosal dissection (ESD) For early gastric neoplasms between high-volume and low-volume centers: multi-center retrospective questionnaire study conducted by the Nagano ESD Study Group. Intern Med 2010;49:253–9.

14. Oyama T, Yahagi N, Ponchon T, et al. How to establish endoscopic submucosal dissection in Western countries. World J Gastroenterol 2015;21:11209–20.

15. Ebigbo A, Probst A, Rommele C, et al. Step-up training for colorectal and gastric ESD and the challenge of ESD training in the proximal colon: results from a German Center. Endosc Int Open 2018;6:E524–30.

16. Hayashi Y, Miura Y, Yamamoto H. Pocket-creation method for the safe, reliable, and efficient endoscopic submucosal dissection of colorectal lateral spreading tumors. Dig Endosc 2015;27:534–5.

17. Toyonaga T, Man IM, Morita Y, et al. Endoscopic submucosal dissection (ESD) versus simplified/hybrid ESD. Gastrointest Endosc Clin N Am 2014;24:191–9.

18. Schmidt A, Bauerfeind P, Gubler C, et al. Endoscopic full-thickness resection in the colorectum with a novel over-the-scope device: first experience. Endoscopy 2015;47:719–25.

19. Marin-Gabriel JC, Diaz-Tasende J, Rodriguez-Munoz S, et al. Colonic endoscopic full-thickness resection (EFTR) with the over-the-scope device (FTRD): a short case series. Rev Esp Enferm Dig 2017;109:230–3.

Underwater Endoscopic Mucosal Resection

Andrew Nett, MD*, Kenneth Binmoeller, MD

KEYWORDS

- UEMR • Underwater endoscopic mucosal resection • Colorectal neoplasm
- Colonic polyps • Residual neoplasm • Water submersion colonoscopy

KEY POINTS

- Purported advantages of submucosal injection before resection have sparse evidential backing. Poorly performed submucosal injection can make EMR more challenging and may increase the risk of certain complications.
- Compared with reported outcomes of conventional EMR, underwater EMR achieves high rates of en bloc resection and low rates of lesion recurrence.
- Water submersion results in mucosal fold involution and separation from the underlying muscularis mucosa, enabling snare entrapment of large colonic lesions while protecting against perforation and transmural thermal injury.

INTRODUCTION

Endoscopic mucosal resection (EMR) has definitively replaced surgical resection in the treatment of large and/or sessile colonic mucosal neoplasms. The standard methodology of EMR involves submucosal injection of fluid, typically saline, for creation of a submucosal cushion that separates superficial lesions from the underlying muscularis propria before resection. The rationale is that the fluid accumulated within the submucosal space protects against full-thickness colonic perforation, lifts overlying sessile flat lesions to facilitate entrapment within a snare, and, by increasing the distance between the electrocautery source and the extramural space, mitigates against transmural thermal injury.[1,2] Submucosal injection also carries the purported benefit of identifying the presence of deeply invading neoplastic tissue, which may be expected to prevent tissue lifting in response to injection (the "nonlifting sign"). This sign is unreliable, however, because submucosal scarring may also cause the absence of tissue lift.

Conventional submucosal injection-assisted EMR has become a well-established standard of practice despite a surprising dearth of studies proving its clinical benefit.

Disclosure Statement: The authors have nothing to disclose.
Interventional Endoscopy Services, California Pacific Medical Center, 1101 Van Ness Ave. Floor 3, San Francisco, CA 94109, USA
* Corresponding author.
E-mail address: nettas@sutterhealth.org

Gastrointest Endoscopy Clin N Am 29 (2019) 659–673
https://doi.org/10.1016/j.giec.2019.05.004
1052-5157/19/Published by Elsevier Inc.

The rationale for this technique has indeed propagated as dogma. In 2015, the American Society of Gastrointestinal Endoscopy Technology Status Evaluation Report emphasized that "the cushion lifts the lesion, facilitating capture and removal by using a snare while minimizing mechanical or electrocautery damage to the deeper layers of the GI wall".[3] Although the historical safety profile of conventional submucosal injection–based EMR seems to lend credence to these theorized advantages, the actual benefit of submucosal saline injection is not well studied. A single in vivo study has analyzed the effect of submucosal saline injection on the depth of thermal tissue injury caused by electrocautery applications in 6 porcine subjects. Although a snare device was not specifically tested, submucosal saline injection was found to have overall equivocal benefit for other monopolar electrocautery techniques, reducing thermal injury in response to argon plasma coagulation (APC) and heat-probe therapy but achieving no reduction in injury because of hot biopsy forceps.[4] In addition, at least for small polyps 5 to 9 mm in size, prospective, randomized comparison of hot snare polypectomy with or without preceding saline/epinephrine injection lift has shown no difference in either complete resection rate or clinical safety.[5]

Apart from its basis on limited evidence behind claims of enhanced safety, conventional saline-injection EMR achieves clinical outcomes that leave room for improvement, specifically when considering reported rates of piecemeal resection and lesion recurrence. Of note, a remarkably high incidence of residual or recurrent neoplasia has been reported after conventional EMR—as high as 15% to 55%.[2,6–8] Of course, if surveillance colonoscopy is performed a short time after initial resection, recurrent lesions may be small and relatively easily resectable. Their occurrence, however, mandates subsequent additional and more frequent surveillance colonoscopy, increasing procedural and financial burden for patients. Occasionally, stubborn recurrent lesions may even eventually require surgical intervention as progressive scarring from repeat endoscopic resection renders complete endoscopic resection more and more difficult and risky. The primary predictors of adenomatous lesion recurrence following conventional EMR are piecemeal resection technique and, likely interrelated, large polyp lesion size (which makes piecemeal resection necessary). When performing conventional EMR, a lesion size greater than 2 cm typically requires piecemeal resection. Snare size and the risk of capturing the muscle layer during snaring limit the ability to perform en bloc resection on larger lesions.[9,10] The presence of residual/recurrent adenomas after conventional EMR is also more likely if neoplasia ablation with APC was performed during initial resection.[10]

The high recurrence rate following piecemeal EMR is a critical weakness, prompting growing favor for endoscopic submucosal dissection (ESD) as a method of en bloc resection of large or flat colonic neoplasia. Per Japanese guidelines, for colon lesions greater than 2 cm with Paris IIc or IIa + IIc morphology, or any lesion greater than 3 cm in size, ESD should be considered as a preferred method of resection. In addition to lesion size, depth of neoplastic involvement may also affect piecemeal resection in conventional EMR. Submucosal invasion may interfere with lift from submucosal injection, and thus may frequently necessitate piecemeal resection during conventional EMR, complicating histologic assessment of R0 or margin-free resection as well as the depth of invasion.[11] As such, given high associated rates of multifocal submucosal invasion, nongranular type lateral spreading tumors are also suggested candidates for ESD. In all of these scenarios, enthusiasm for ESD rests on the ability for en bloc removal when it cannot be achieved by conventional EMR. The higher en bloc resection rates of ESD, however, are accompanied by a significantly higher rate of perforation.[12] Compared with conventional EMR, ESD is a time-consuming, cumbersome, and costly technique with increased complication risk. The learning curve of traditional

ESD may be steep, especially in the right colon where ease of positioning and colonoscope responsiveness are diminished.[11] Specialized accessories make ESD more expensive than conventional EMR. In combination, the cost, procedure length, and technical difficulty are prohibitive practical barriers to the widespread dissemination of ESD. Thus, both conventional EMR and ESD fall short as resection methodologies.

UNDERWATER ENDOSCOPIC MUCOSAL RESECTION

Water submersion during colonoscopy (the "underwater" technique) enhances several outcomes. Compared with the conventional gas-insufflation technique, underwater exchange results in decreased sedation needs, improved patient comfort, and higher adenoma detection rates, as demonstrated by multiple randomized controlled trials.[13–19] Diagnostic yield may also be improved because water has a focus and magnification effect that improves lesion resolution, which helps to define lesion margins under white light or narrow-band imaging.[20] In a gas-insufflated colon, lesions may be hidden within deep valleys concealed by folds, but underwater these lesions can be revealed as they float into view.

This underwater floating effect is lucidly demonstrated with endoscopic ultrasonography (EUS). In fact, observations during endosonography that with water submersion the mucosa and submucosa float away from the muscularis propria instigated the development of the UEMR technique by Binmoeller and colleagues.[21] Removal of intraluminal air decreases colonic wall tension, permitting the wall to reassume its normal thickness in a collapsed state. Underwater, the fat density of the submucosa creates tissue buoyancy, lifting the overlying mucosa and any mucosal lesions away from the muscularis propria. As such, when the colon is filled with water, the muscularis propria continues to act as a circular frame of the colon while the mucosa and submucosa drift away from the muscle, forming multiple involutions similar to the rugal folds of the stomach (**Fig. 1**). These mechanics serve to separate adenomatous mucosal lesions from the muscularis propria without the need for submucosal injection. The wall-layer separation that occurs enables snare entrapment of superficial lesions, limiting concern for inadvertent capture of the muscularis and resultant immediate perforation. Intraluminal water also protects against deep thermal injury by acting as a heat sink. This heat-sink effect, coupled with the increased distance between colon wall layers, may decrease the risk of full-thickness and transmural thermal injury, protecting against postpolypectomy electrocautery syndrome as well as delayed perforation.[22]

Binmoeller and colleagues[21] first shared the efficacy and safety of UEMR in 2012. In the initial published series, 62 large sessile benign colorectal lesions (>2 cm in size, mean size 34 mm) were removed with 100% therapeutic efficacy using UEMR over a period of slightly less than a year. Promising low rates of lesion recurrence were apparent from the beginning. Surveillance colonoscopy, performed 3 months after initial resection with biopsies of the resection-site scar as well as any suspicious tissue, showed possible recurrent adenoma in only 1.9% with 90% adherence to follow-up. In the sole case, possible recurrence consisted of a 5-mm adenomatous nodule adjacent to the prior site of resection at a tethered fold, which may have been either a true recurrence or a missed residual satellite lesion. The safety profile was also favorable. Delayed bleeding occurred in 5% of patients while perforation occurred in none. Clip closure of the resection wound had been performed when feasible, in 27% of resections.

Since this initial publication, multiple successive prospective series and one cohort study have reinforced the efficacy and success of colonic UEMR. In 2014, Wang and

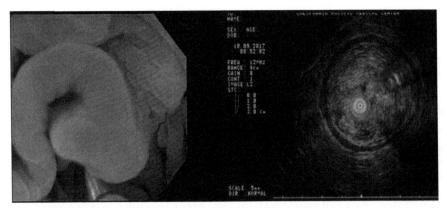

Fig. 1. Underwater, the mucosa and submucosa involute while the muscularis propria maintains a circular conformation.

colleagues[7] published a series of 43 lesions averaging 20 mm in size. They achieved complete resection for 98% of lesions with the caveat that the hot biopsy forceps stripping technique was applied for islands of residual lesion in 11.6% of cases, particularly with lesions of larger size ($P = .001$). These investigators also relied on APC for residual neoplastic islands in 16.3% of cases, whereas the initial published series by Binmoeller and colleagues[21] used no thermal ablation therapy. In the sole case of residual lesion, endoscopic resection was terminated after the lesion was noted to involve the appendiceal orifice. Delayed bleeding occurred in 1 patient after simultaneous removal of a 6-cm tubulovillous adenoma and a 1-cm cecal tubular adenoma. No perforation or postpolypectomy syndrome occurred. In 2015, Uedo and colleagues[23] were the next to publish on the efficacy and safety of UEMR, presenting a series involving 11 consecutive patients with a mean lesion size of 19 mm. They reported 100% successful complete resection without complications. In the same year, a larger prospective series by Curcio and colleagues[24] also demonstrated a 100% complete resection rate with no complications and 0% recurrence at 3-month follow-up for a total of 72 consecutive patients with 81 polyps.

Overall, more than 500 cases of colonic UEMR have been reported (**Table 1**). In these prospective series and cohort publications delayed bleeding rates have occurred at a rate of 0.5% to 6.7%, with 1 case requiring blood transfusions and 2 reported instances of pursuit of colonoscopy for hemostatic intervention.[1,2] A recent meta-analysis performed by Spadaccini and colleagues[29] reviews UEMR outcomes of 508 lesions resected in 433 patients. Including 7 prospective series and 3 retrospective series, the pooled rate of complete resection was 96.36% with a mean recurrence rate of 8.82% occurring over a surveillance period of 7.7 months (range 4–15 months). These outcomes were noted despite inclusion of more difficult target lesions, including recurrent adenomas with scarring following prior piecemeal resection and lesions located at the appendiceal orifice. The pooled rate of delayed bleeding was 2.85%. No perforations occurred. The series published by Kawamura and colleagues[28] in 2018, also referenced in **Table 1**, did include a single case of perforation following underwater resection, but submucosal injection was actually performed before UEMR in this case. Ponogoti and Rex[30] describe the only reported case of perforation caused by a strictly UEMR technique. These investigators specified that the UEMR was performed in a retroflexed position, suggesting that the retroflexed scope stretched and thinned the colonic wall, negating the typical protective effect of water immersion and its associated collapsed colonic wall state.

Table 1
Published experience of underwater endoscopic mucosal resection (UEMR)

UEMR Series	No. of Lesions	Size (Mean, mm)	Endoscopic Complete Resection (%)	Piecemeal Resection (%)	Biopsy Forceps Stripping	APC	Residual/ Recurrent Lesion (%)	Follow-up (Median, wk)	Clip Closure (%)	Delayed Bleeding (%)	Perforation (%)	Postpoly-pectomy Syndrome (%)	EUS (%)	Resection Time (Median, min)
Binmoeller et al,[21] 2012	62	33.8	100	NR	Yes	No	1.90	15.2	27	5	0	0	100	18
Wang et al,[7] 2014	43	20	97.70	NR	Yes, 11.6%	Yes, 16.3%	NR	NR	23.30	2.30	0	0	4.70	12.7 (mean)
Uedo et al,[23] 2015	11	19	100	45	No	No	NR	NR	NR	0	0	NR	0	NR
Curcio et al,[24] 2015	81	18.7	100	32	No	No	0	48	40.70	0	0	0	11	7
Binmoeller et al,[25] 2015	53	30	100	45	No	No	4.70	31	0	2	0	0	100	3
Amato et al,[26] 2016	25	24.6	100	24	No	No	9.10	24	0	0	0	NR	0	13
Schenck et al,[1] 2017	73	25.4	99	52	Yes	Yes	7.3	23.2	0	4.10	0	0	0	NR
Siau et al,[27] 2018[a]	97	25	99	55	No	Yes, 13.4%	13.60	16	35.60	2	0	0	0	NR
Kawamura et al,[28] 2018	64	16.2	100	19	No	No	NR	NR	NR	4.69	1.57[b]	0	4.69	NR

Abbreviations: APC, argon plasma coagulation; EUS, endoscopic ultrasonography; NR, not recorded.
[a] 29.9% of resections in this study were actually performed with saline injection before underwater resection.
[b] Perforation occurred in 1 case in this study, but occurred during the only resection for which submucosal injection was first performed.
Data from Refs.[1,7,21,23–28]

UNDERWATER ENDOSCOPIC MUCOSAL RESECTION TECHNIQUE

An adult high-definition single-channel colonoscope accompanied by an auxiliary water jet is the ideal scope choice for UEMR (CF-H180AL; Olympus Corp. of the Americas, Center Valley, PA). Compared with a pediatric colonoscope, the adult colonoscope has near focus capability, which sharpens underwater images. An accessory cap (Model D-201-15004; Olympus) aids in scope tip stabilization and may be used to flatten folds and mechanically tamponade bleeding vessels. Glucagon administration is typically avoided in order to take advantage of colon wall contractions to induce prolapse of large lesions into the resection snare. Although water-exchange intubation should be pursued for added advantages of lesion detection and patient comfort, if the lesion is located under gas insufflation, gas should first be removed from the target colonic segment. Sterile room-temperature water is then infused (generally 100–300 mL) until the lesion is fully submersed. Adequate water infusion is important: Amato and colleagues[26] have noted an association between insufficient initial water infusion and postresection bleeding, attributed to poor polyp flotation.

Lesion inspection with both high-definition white light and narrow-band imaging underwater then identifies the presence of any concerning pit and vascular patterns. If features suggestive of malignancy exist (type IIc Paris morphology, Kudo type V pit pattern, NICE type 3 characteristics), EUS is performed to help exclude deeply invasive disease.[2,7,11] Following confirmation of resectability appropriateness the perimeter of a lesion is routinely marked, as cautery artifact created during resection may obfuscate identification of residual adenomatous change. Demarcation of the lesion margins is performed by applying APC 1 to 2 mm away from the perimeter of the lesion. For precision, the 7F probe tip is applied directly to the mucosa, briefly delivering energy using 0.8 L/min flow at 30 W. In this manner, the APC creates round dots of coagulum that are readily identified during resection (**Fig. 2**).

Next a stiff, braided snare is used to perform resection under complete water submersion. En bloc resection being the goal, snare selection is guided by lesion size such that the open snare encompasses the entire lesion when possible. After opening the snare, it is positioned completely around the demarcated lesion margins. Pressing the snare against the colon wall induces the adenoma and surrounding mucosa through the snare orifice (**Fig. 3**). A "torque and crimp" technique is applied: subtle to-and-fro movement of the snare catheter coupled with gentle water suction and torquing of the scope will crimp the lesion and a rim of surrounding normal tissue to secure lesion entrapment.

Ongoing water infusion to maintain and enhance visualization is tempting during this process, but excessive infusion during snare entrapment should be avoided because the water jet drives the mucosa and submucosa back up against the muscularis, possibly risking either incomplete resection or perforation resulting from muscle entrapment. Excessive suctioning may also be dangerous, resulting in involution of the full thickness of the colon wall through the snare with consequent perforation after resection.[6] When larger lesions remain expanded beyond the size of the snare orifice, patience is a virtue, as infolding of the mucosa and the submucosa that occurs during eventual colonic contraction can often enable complete lesion capture and en bloc resection.

Once the lesion is fully entrapped, uninterrupted electrocautery current is delivered while steady and continuous closing pressure is applied to the snare. The authors typically use a blended current (DRYCUT, effect 5, 60W, VIO 300D; Erbe, Tübingen, Germany), but preferentially use a pure cutting current in locations where the bowel

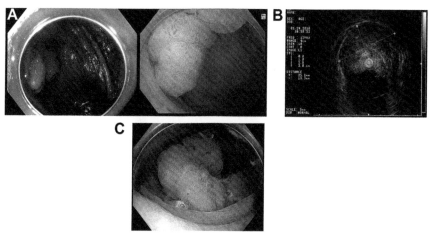

Fig. 2. Lesion visualization and demarcation. (*A*) The lesion contracts and floats into the lumen following air removal followed by water immersion. (*B*) Endosonography confirms the presence of no deeply invasive disease. (*C*) Diathermic markings are made to demarcate the lesion margin.

wall is thin or heavy scarring is present (AUTOCUT, effect 5, 80W, VIO 300D; Erbe). To enhance the potential heat-sink effect of water submersion, water is continuously infused during application of the electrocautery current. As with other methods of snare resection, care must be taken to not skim across lesions at an inadequate depth, especially when scar tissue exists.

Immediate bleeding is treated by directly grasping and cauterizing vessels with a coagulation (Swift Coag 50W, VIO 300D; Erbe). The benefit of prophylactically coagulating vessels is unclear, but large vessels exposed within the resection bed may also be treated using coagulation forceps.[31] Inspection for residual perimeter markings or adenomatous tissue determines whether any further resection should be performed with additional snaring (**Fig. 4**). Hot biopsy forceps stripping may be performed to remove any remnant adenoma when necessary.

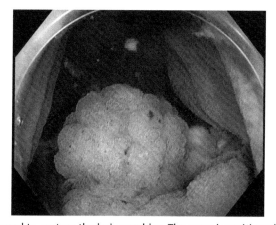

Fig. 3. A snare is used to capture the lesion en bloc. The snare is positioned such that it captures the lesion and its surrounding diathermic markings.

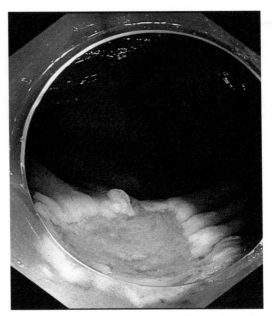

Fig. 4. Examination of the resection site following en bloc underwater resection. No residual diathermic markings are present, consistent with complete resection.

Follow-up surveillance colonoscopy should be conducted to confirm complete, curative resection. In general, colonoscopy should be considered 6 to 12 months following initial resection to assess for the presence of residual or recurrent lesions. This time frame is based on prior study showing that 91% of recurrent adenomas occur within 6 months and 98% develop by 12 months.[32] Following conventional EMR, biopsies of inconspicuous-appearing resection-site scars yielded histologic evidence of residual/recurrent adenoma in 16 of 228 (7%) cases in a 2-center study from Germany (with a total recurrent/residual rate of 32%).[33] Although the anticipated rate of recurrent/residual lesions may be anticipated to be less following UEMR, given the possibility of microscopic recurrence the authors recommend taking multiple biopsies of the scar site, even if no grossly endoscopic recurrence is visualized.

ADVANTAGES OVER CONVENTIONAL ENDOSCOPIC MUCOSAL RESECTION

As discussed previously, the rationale for submucosal injection before resection is backed with surprisingly little science. As opposed to conventional EMR, the colon wall is under reduced tension and submucosal injection is unnecessary during UEMR, which may confer several theoretic advantages. While conventional EMR rests on the tenet that a cushion of submucosal fluid is necessary to protect against deep wall injury, the perforation rates observed during UEMR seem comparable with or lower than the published rate of 0.5% to 0.8% that occurs during conventional EMR.[12] The act of submucosal injection may also actually increase perforation risk if misdirected. As observed directly during peroral endoscopic myotomy, the connective tissue between the inner circular and outer longitudinal layers of the muscularis propria can be expanded with fluid injection, leading to muscle splitting. During colon EMR, inadvertent deep injection into the connective tissue separating the circular and longitudinal muscle layers may result in muscle-layer capture and at least partial-thickness defect after resection. This unrecognized technical error may explain why muscularis propria is sometimes noted within resection specimen pathology. Even deeper misdirected injection may also cause complications that may be avoided altogether with UEMR. With inadvertent transcolonic tattoo injection, several complications may occur including peritonitis, perforation, abscess development, and formation of an inflammatory pseudotumor. Of course, these complications may be specific to an inflammatory reaction to tattoo ink. Transcolonic submucosal fluid injection of any kind, however, should not automatically be taken as inconsequential. Although transmural thermal injury from electrocautery is blamed for postpolypectomy syndrome, it is also conceivable that transmural injection of fluid by a needle introduced through the unsterile colon lumen could cause clinically significant transient extramural inflammation.

The reported high rates of neoplasia recurrence after conventional EMR insinuate other potential harm caused by submucosal injection. Presumably recurrent growth results from unintentional incomplete resection, but an alternative explanation may be neoplastic seeding caused by submucosal injection. Needle-tract seeding is a real occurrence in several endoscopic scenarios. EUS-guided fine-needle aspiration (EUS-FNA) may cause seeding of the gastrointestinal (GI) wall during sampling of various tumor types.[34] In the instance of hepatocellular carcinoma, a 2.7% overall incidence of needle-tract tumor seeding after biopsy has been reported by a systematic review.[35] An increased risk of peritoneal metastases is also associated with prior transperitoneal biopsy of hilar cholangiocarcinoma.[36] In fact, a history of EUS-FNA of hilar cholangiocarcinoma can make patients ineligible for liver transplantation because of consternation over FNA-related tumor seeding. Potential tumor seeding has also been reported as a consequence of unintentional perforation during endoscopic resection.[37] Although rates may vary, perforation may of course occur with any resection methodology but, given that needle-tract seeding is a known phenomenon, one cannot overlook putative deeper spread of neoplastic cells into the submucosa during submucosal injection. UEMR, by avoiding submucosal injection altogether, eliminates concern for such a risk.

Apart from introducing these proposed risks, submucosal injection can also technically complicate snare resection in several ways. Usually submucosal injection lifts a sessile or flat lesion relative to surrounding normal tissue. Fluid can at times dissipate quickly and/or preferentially to the perilesional area, however, which results in paradoxic flattening or relative depression of the lesion and increased difficulty of snare entrapment. Submucosal expansion may also increase the tissue tension of the overlying surface, hindering snare grasp of the mucosa with resultant slippage and lesion scraping during snare closure. Poor injection execution may impair lesion access by either displacing the lesion into a partially concealed position or cramping the lumen and restricting maneuverability with an oversized submucosal bulge. Needle puncture and injection into the submucosa also will occasionally precipitate bleeding or induce colonic contraction with resultant reduced visibility. Finally, by increasing the lesion area, piecemeal rather than en bloc resection may become necessary following injection.

Although the underwater technique creates many theoretic technical and safety advantages that obviate submucosal injection, enhanced ability for en bloc resection of larger lesions may be the most important and substantiated improvement over conventional EMR. UEMR has been shown to increase the efficacy of resection of larger lesions compared with conventional EMR. Underwater, the colon mucosa and submucosa are contracted and involuted. Large mucosal lesions thus occupy a diminished projected area along the colon wall compared with the expanded footprint they have when the mucosa and submucosa are flattened and stretched against the muscularis by air insufflation. Thus, a resection snare with a fixed maximum size can capture involuted underwater lesions with a surface area that is actually much larger than the area of the snare's orifice. In a prospective series involving UEMR of 53 larger lateral spreading tumors with a median size of 30 mm (20–40 mm), en bloc resection was achieved in 55% of cases with use of a 33-mm polypectomy snare.[25] Despite tackling larger lesions en bloc, complications remained low with a delayed bleeding rate of 4% and absence of any perforations. At 31-week median follow-up (range 7–71 weeks), residual adenoma was found in 5% of cases during surveillance colonoscopy.

The real promise of enhanced en bloc resection rates is the aforementioned link between piecemeal resection and lesion recurrence. Although no prospective, comparative data are yet published to establish reduced rates of lesion recurrence following UEMR versus conventional EMR, a retrospective comparison of these methodologies for the treatment of large polyps does suggest a difference in outcomes.[1] In 2017, Schenck and colleagues[1] reported a higher rate of complete macroscopic resection achieved with UEMR compared with conventional EMR in lesions $\geq$15 mm (98.6% vs 87.1%, P = .012) as well as lower associated rates of adenomatous recurrence (7.3% vs 28.3% at initial follow-up, odds ratio 5.0). No difference in complication rates was present. In the meta-analysis by Spadaccini and colleagues,[29] pooled outcomes of UEMR confirm high rates of en bloc resection coupled with low rates of lesion recurrence.

Authoritative comparison of UEMR and conventional EMR in the form of a randomized controlled trial (RCT) is not yet available. An international multicenter RCT comparing submucosal injection-assisted with UEMR has presented interim results, however, consisting of data from 210 large colonic lateral spreading tumors.[38] UEMR resulted in a significantly higher en bloc resection rate (51% vs 25%, P = .001) with need for significantly fewer adjunct ablative techniques (11% vs 26%, P = .006). The mean lesion size was 28.5 mm and was statistically equivalent in each treatment arm. Residual lesions were noted on follow-up in 3.4% of UEMR cases versus 10% in conventional EMR cases (P = .272). Interim analysis in the RCT conducted by Hamerski and colleagues[38] also showed another potential advantage of UEMR, which resulted in significantly shorter resection and total procedure times compared with conventional EMR (10.2 vs 18.4 min [P<.0001] and 37.5 vs 44.2 min [P = .035], respectively).

Numerous studies have now demonstrated UEMR en bloc resection rates of more than 50% for colonic lesions greater than 2 cm. The technique outperforms conventional EMR in this regard, and undermines current societal guidelines recommending conventional piecemeal resection or ESD of lesions this size.[11,39] There are several additional clinical scenarios beyond large polyp size in which conventional EMR is contraindicated or avoided, but UEMR has established efficacy and safety. Specifically, UEMR may be advantageous for lesions located at the ileocecal valve, appendiceal orifice, colonic anastomoses, or in the presence of significant scarring that prevents submucosal lift.

Conventional EMR is technically demanding at the ileocecal valve, where there is a higher risk of incomplete resection and perforation. The authors have reported outcomes on UEMR in a prospective series of 91 consecutive laterally spreading tumors involving the ileocecal valve. Complete resection was achieved in 98% of cases (25% en bloc rate with median lesion size of 25 mm). The delayed bleeding rate was 9% and no perforations occurred. The rate of residual adenoma was 1.7% at median 25-week follow-up, although surveillance data were only available for 59% of patients.[40]

At the appendiceal orifice, a thin wall and lack of muscularis propria at appendix insertion augment perforation risk and make conventional EMR technically. The appendix can partially evert into the cecal lumen under water submersion. As reported from the authors' center, in a series of 27 consecutive patients, 89% successful resection was achieved using UEMR technique, with 59% of lesions being resected en bloc. The median resection time was 3 minutes. While postpolypectomy syndrome occurred in 7% of cases, no other instances of complications occurred (perforation, appendicitis, or bleeding requiring transfusion). Over a median follow-up of 29 weeks (12–139 weeks), 10% of patients (n = 2) had residual adenoma present.[41]

Scar tissue, often unfortunately iatrogenic, may commonly complicate colon lesion resection. Scarring may develop from prior mucosal biopsies or submucosal tattoo placement, both of which are typically unnecessary if referral to an advanced endoscopist is pursued. Unsuccessful prior EMR attempts may also leave significant scar tissue making lesion resection substantially more difficult by diminishing the ability of a snare to grasp tissue. The snare may repeatedly slip off and over a lesion during closure, causing progressive abrasion of the lesion. It may also interfere with lesion lifting, yielding a false positive "negative lift sign." During injection, the lift of normal surrounding mucosa may actually result in burying and the scarred lesion. As an alternative to EMR, ESD can also be difficult and risky when submucosal fibrosis is present due to tacking of the lesion to the underlying muscularis propria by scar tissue. UEMR is a valuable and potentially superior technique to apply to recurrent lesions. In a comparison of UEMR to repeat conventional EMR for laterally spreading tumors greater than 2 cm in size recurring after prior conventional piecemeal resection, UEMR resulted in higher rates of en bloc resection, complete resection, fewer subsequent adenoma recurrences, and decreased need for APC ablation. In fact, UEMR enabled en bloc resection of recurrent adenoma in ~50% of cases, which is comparable with the rate published for ESD, but with no perforations.[6,42]

ADVANTAGES OVER ENDOSCOPIC SUBMUCOSAL DISSECTION

A prospective, randomized comparison or UEMR and ESD has not been published. In assessment of UEMR versus ESD, however, contrast exists in the reported complication rate, procedure time, and ease of performance. Reported perforation rates of ESD for colon polypectomy may range from 2% to 14%.[12] In addition to its associated high perforation risk, ESD is also technically demanding and arduous, uses additional costly accessories, and requires prolonged training for proper skill development even among seasoned endoscopists.[2,26,43,44] In contradistinction, for endoscopists experienced in the conventional EMR technique, UEMR may be swiftly grasped and is translatable to the community setting, where it has been performed effectively and safely.[1,7,26]

DRAWBACKS OF UNDERWATER ENDOSCOPIC MUCOSAL RESECTION

In the setting of poor bowel preparation, underwater endoscopy can be challenging because of poor visualization. Robust water exchange can improve views but may be time consuming. Although the nonlifting sign may be unreliable, an endoscopist who customarily uses it as a predictor of invasive disease may be frustrated that such information is not available during UEMR. Available data demonstrate that benign adenomas with associated submucosal fibrosis may not lift whereas those with invasive cancer may do so. A multicenter study has shown that endoscopic diagnosis is more reliable than the nonlifting sign; in 10 of 26 lesions with cancer invading beyond 1000 μm into the submucosa, there was false-negative nonlifting sign.[45] The inability to use the nonlifting sign in lesion assessment is a poor reason to cling to conventional EMR. If submucosal lifting is initiated, it can be difficult to shift to UEMR mid-procedure because the submucosal fluid changes the normal buoyancy of the tissue and further restricts working space within the collapsed colon lumen.

ADDITIONAL APPLICATIONS OF UNDERWATER ENDOSCOPIC MUCOSAL RESECTION

The advantages of UEMR are applicable throughout the GI tract. Wall-layer behavior underwater can be exploited at any location where a thin GI wall presents increased potential for perforation. The authors have demonstrated the benefits of UEMR during resection of large duodenal adenomas (median size 35 mm) as well as ampullary adenomas.[46,47]

SUMMARY

Conventional EMR rests on the premise that injection of fluid into the mucosa facilitates snare capture of colonic lesions and mitigates the risk of perforation and transmural thermal injury by separating the target lesion and underlying muscularis propria with a submucosal cushion of fluid. The presumed benefits of submucosal injection, however, have not been proven. Misguided submucosal injection can actually make resection more difficult and potentially riskier. Several lesion characteristics make resection using the conventional EMR technique more complicated. Scarring form prior lesion biopsy, adjacent tattoo placement, or previous failed or incomplete attempts at resection all interfere with submucosal lifting, as well as en bloc and complete resection. Lesion location at the ileocecal valve and appendiceal orifice also is considered to enhance the technical difficulty and complication potential for conventional EMR. As such, these lesions are often referred for surgical resection. In addition to flimsy support behind its theoretic advantages, conventional EMR outcomes fall short. Substantially high lesion recurrence occurs following conventional EMR, which is, in part, likely related to a need for piecemeal resection of most lesions larger than 2 cm. Although colonic ESD may achieve better en bloc resection rates, it can be time consuming and expensive, and carries an increased perforation rate. Its inherent technical complexity is a barrier to widespread uptake. Alternatively, the behavior of colonic mucosal lesions underwater allows UEMR to overcome several of the challenges and shortcomings of conventional EMR. UEMR has been established as an effective, safe, easily learned technique for colon resection. UEMR achieves high rates of en bloc resection, quick resection times, and low rates of lesion recurrence while maintaining an excellent safety profile. Forthcoming RCTs comparing UEMR with conventional EMR may substantiate the promising results established by existing observational studies.

REFERENCES

1. Schenck RJ, Jahann DA, Patrie JT, et al. Underwater endoscopic mucosal resection is associated with fewer recurrences and earlier curative resections compared to conventional endoscopic mucosal resection for large colorectal polyps. Surg Endosc 2017;31(10):4174–83.
2. Gaglia A, Sarkar S. Evaluation and long-term outcomes of the different modalities used in colonic endoscopic mucosal resection. Ann Gastroenterol 2017;30(2): 145–51.

Underwater Endoscopic Mucosal Resection 671

3. ASGE Technology Committee, Goodman AJ, Melson J, Aslanian HR, et al. Endoscopic mucosal resection. Gastrointest Endosc 2015;82(2):215–26.

4. Norton ID, Wang L, Levine SA, et al. Efficacy of colonic submucosal saline solution injection for the reduction of iatrogenic thermal injury. Gastrointest Endosc 2002;56(1):95–9.

5. Kim HS, Jung HY, Park HJ, et al. Hot snare polypectomy with or without saline solution/epinephrine lift for the complete resection of small colorectal polyps. Gastrointest Endosc 2018;87(6):1539–47.

6. Kim HG, Thosani N, Banerjee S, et al. Underwater endoscopic mucosal resection for recurrences after previous piecemeal resection of colorectal polyps (with video). Gastrointest Endosc 2014;80(6):1094–102.

7. Wang AY, Flynn MM, Patrie JT, et al. Underwater endoscopic mucosal resection of colorectal neoplasia is easily learned, efficacious, and safe. Surg Endosc 2014; 28(4):1348–54.

8. Fukami N, Lee JH. Endoscopic treatment of large sessile and flat colorectal lesions. Curr Opin Gastroenterol 2006;22(1):54–9.

9. Woodward TA, Heckman MG, Cleveland P, et al. Predictors of complete endoscopic mucosal resection of flat and depressed gastrointestinal neoplasia of the colon. Am J Gastroenterol 2012;107(5):650–4.

10. Moss A, Williams SJ, Hourigan LF, et al. Long-term adenoma recurrence following wide-field endoscopic mucosal resection (WF-EMR) for advanced colonic mucosal neoplasia is infrequent: results and risk factors in 1000 cases from the Australian Colonic EMR (ACE) study. Gut 2015;64(1):57–65.

11. Tanaka S, Kashida H, Saito Y, et al. JGES guidelines for colorectal endoscopic submucosal dissection/endoscopic mucosal resection. Dig Endosc 2015;27(4): 417–34.

12. Nakajima T, Saito Y, Tanaka S, et al. Current status of endoscopic resection strategy for large, early colorectal neoplasia in Japan. Surg Endosc 2013;27(9): 3262–70.

13. Jia H, Pan Y, Guo X, et al. Water exchange method significantly improves adenoma detection rate: a multicenter, randomized controlled trial. Am J Gastroenterol 2017;112(4):568–76.

14. Cadoni S, Falt P, Rondonotti E, et al. Water exchange for screening colonoscopy increases adenoma detection rate: a multicenter, double-blinded, randomized controlled trial. Endoscopy 2017;49(5):456–67.

15. Hsieh YH, Tseng CW, Hu CT, et al. Prospective multicenter randomized controlled trial comparing adenoma detection rate in colonoscopy using water exchange, water immersion, and air insufflation. Gastrointest Endosc 2017;86(1):192–201.

16. Cadoni S, Falt P, Gallittu P, et al. Impact of carbon dioxide insufflation and water exchange on postcolonoscopy outcomes in patients receiving on-demand sedation: a randomized controlled trial. Gastrointest Endosc 2017;85(1):210–8.e1.

17. Cadoni S, Falt P, Gallittu P, et al. Water exchange is the least painful colonoscope insertion technique and increases completion of unsedated colonoscopy. Clin Gastroenterol Hepatol 2015;13(11):1972–80.e1-3.

18. Hsieh YH, Koo M, Leung FW. A patient-blinded randomized, controlled trial comparing air insufflation, water immersion, and water exchange during minimally sedated colonoscopy. Am J Gastroenterol 2014;109(9):1390–400.

19. Cadoni S, Gallittu P, Sanna S, et al. A two-center randomized controlled trial of water-aided colonoscopy versus air insufflation colonoscopy. Endoscopy 2014; 46(3):212–8.

20. Cammarota G, Cesaro P, Cazzato A, et al. The water immersion technique is easy to learn for routine use during EGD for duodenal villous evaluation: a single-center 2-year experience. J Clin Gastroenterol 2009;43(3):244–8.

21. Binmoeller KF, Weilert F, Shah J, et al. "Underwater" EMR without submucosal injection for large sessile colorectal polyps (with video). Gastrointest Endosc 2012; 75(5):1086–91.

22. Hsieh Y, Binmoeller KF, Leung FW. Su1664 underwater polypectomy: heat-sink effect in an experimental model. Gastrointest Endosc 2016;83(5):1.

23. Uedo N, Nemeth A, Johansson GW, et al. Underwater endoscopic mucosal resection of large colorectal lesions. Endoscopy 2015;47(2):172–4.

24. Curcio G, Granata A, Ligresti D, et al. Underwater colorectal EMR: remodeling endoscopic mucosal resection. Gastrointest Endosc 2015;81(5):1238–42.

25. Binmoeller KF, Hamerski CM, Shah JN, et al. Attempted underwater en bloc resection for large (2-4 cm) colorectal laterally spreading tumors (with video). Gastrointest Endosc 2015;81(3):713–8.

26. Amato A, Radaelli F, Spinzi G. Underwater endoscopic mucosal resection: The third way for en bloc resection of colonic lesions? United Eur Gastroenterol J 2016;4(4):595–8.

27. Siau K, Ishaq S, Cadoni S, et al. Feasibility and outcomes of underwater endoscopic mucosal resection for ≥10 mm colorectal polyps. Surg Endosc 2018; 32(6):2656–63.

28. Kawamura T, Sakai H, Ogawa T, et al. Feasibility of underwater endoscopic mucosal resection for colorectal lesions: a single center study in Japan. Gastroenterol Res 2018;11(4):274–9.

29. Spadaccini M, Fuccio L, Lamonaca L, et al. Underwater EMR for colorectal lesions: a systematic review with meta-analysis (with video). Gastrointest Endosc 2019;89(6):1109–16.e4.

30. Ponugoti PL, Rex DK. Perforation during underwater EMR. Gastrointest Endosc 2016;84(3):543–4.

31. Yoon JY, Kim JH, Lee JY, et al. Clinical outcomes for patients with perforations during endoscopic submucosal dissection of laterally spreading tumors of the colorectum. Surg Endosc 2013;27(2):487–93.

32. Belderbos TD, Leenders M, Moons LM, et al. Local recurrence after endoscopic mucosal resection of nonpedunculated colorectal lesions: systematic review and meta-analysis. Endoscopy 2014;46(5):388–402.

33. Knabe M, Pohl J, Gerges C, et al. Standardized long-term follow-up after endoscopic resection of large, nonpedunculated colorectal lesions: a prospective two-center study. Am J Gastroenterol 2014;109(2):183–9.

34. Yokoyama K, Ushio J, Numao N, et al. Esophageal seeding after endoscopic ultrasound-guided fine-needle aspiration of a mediastinal tumor. Endosc Int Open 2017;5(9):E913–7.

35. Silva MA, Hegab B, Hyde C, et al. Needle track seeding following biopsy of liver lesions in the diagnosis of hepatocellular cancer: a systematic review and meta-analysis. Gut 2008;57(11):1592–6.

36. Heimbach JK, Sanchez W, Rosen CB, et al. Trans-peritoneal fine needle aspiration biopsy of hilar cholangiocarcinoma is associated with disease dissemination. HPB (Oxford) 2011;13(5):356–60.

37. Gleeson FC, Lee JH, Dewitt JM. Tumor seeding associated with selected gastrointestinal endoscopic interventions. Clin Gastroenterol Hepatol 2018;16(9): 1385–8.

38. Hamerski CM, Wang AY, Amato A, et al. 121 injection-assisted versus underwater endoscopic mucosal resection without injection for the treatment of colorectal laterally spreading tumors: interim analysis of an international multicenter randomized controlled trial. Gastrointest Endosc 2018;87(6):AB55–6.
39. Ferlitsch M, Moss A, Hassan C, et al. Colorectal polypectomy and endoscopic mucosal resection (EMR): European Society of Gastrointestinal Endoscopy (ESGE) clinical guideline. Endoscopy 2017;49(3):270–97.
40. Levy I, Hamerski CM, Nett AS, et al. Su1618 underwater endoscopic mucosal resection (UEMR) of laterally spreading tumors involving the ileocecal valve. Gastrointest Endosc 2017;85(5):1.
41. Binmoeller KF, Hamerski CM, Shah JN, et al. Underwater EMR of adenomas of the appendiceal orifice (with video). Gastrointest Endosc 2016;83(3):638–42.
42. Sakamoto T, Matsuda T, Otake Y, et al. Predictive factors of local recurrence after endoscopic piecemeal mucosal resection. J Gastroenterol 2012;47(6):635–40.
43. Uraoka T, Parra-Blanco A, Yahagi N. Colorectal endoscopic submucosal dissection: is it suitable in western countries? J Gastroenterol Hepatol 2013;28(3):406–14.
44. Saito Y, Uraoka T, Yamaguchi Y, et al. A prospective, multicenter study of 1111 colorectal endoscopic submucosal dissections (with video). Gastrointest Endosc 2010;72(6):1217–25.
45. Kobayashi N, Saito Y, Sano Y, et al. Determining the treatment strategy for colorectal neoplastic lesions: endoscopic assessment or the non-lifting sign for diagnosing invasion depth? Endoscopy 2007;39(8):701–5.
46. Binmoeller KF, Shah JN, Bhat YM, et al. "Underwater" EMR of sporadic laterally spreading nonampullary duodenal adenomas (with video). Gastrointest Endosc 2013;78(3):496–502.
47. Binmoeller K, Kato M, Shah JN, et al. Mo1451 "Underwater" ampullectomy for benign adenomas: prospective study of a novel technique. Gastrointest Endosc 2013;77(5):1.

Surgery Versus Endoscopic Mucosal Resection Versus Endoscopic Submucosal Dissection for Large Polyps

Making Sense of When to Use Which Approach

Norio Fukami, MD

KEYWORDS

- ESD (endoscopic submucosal dissection) • EMR (endoscopic mucosal resection)
- Large colon polyps • TAMIS (transanal minimally invasive surgery)
- TEMS (transanal endoscopic microsurgery)

KEY POINTS

- Endoscopic resection is highly effective and less costly than surgery. It should be the gold standard for large premalignant colorectal lesions.
- Lesion assessment would allow proper selection of treatment of large colorectal lesions. It is important to assess for the presence of invasive cancer during the endoscopic examination and to predict the depth of invasion by endoscopic features associated with deep submucosal invasion.
- Primary endoscopic resection (ER) with proper handling of tissue is beneficial for suspected high-grade dysplasia and early-stage cancer. ER of malignant lesions was reported to not affect surgical outcomes.
- High-quality endoscopic mucosal resection is highly effective for large colorectal lesions but requires close surveillance and additional treatments.
- Endoscopic submucosal dissection (ESD) offers lower recurrence of lesions and higher en bloc and margin negative resections, especially for lesions with concerning features of invasive cancer. Proper application of ESD is likely cost-effective and beneficial for certain patients who can avoid invasive surgical treatment.

INTRODUCTION

Endoscopic resection (ER) of colorectal lesions has led to the reduction of incidence and mortality of colorectal cancer. ER is effective therapy for premalignant complex polyps and is more cost-effective compared with surgery.[1,2]

Disclosure: The author has received consultant fees from Boston Scientific, Olympus America, and Lumendi.
Division of Gastroenterology and Hepatology, Mayo Clinic College of Medicine and Science, Mayo Clinic Arizona, 13400 East Shea Boulevard, Scottsdale, AZ 85259, USA
E-mail address: fukami.norio@mayo.edu

Gastrointest Endoscopy Clin N Am 29 (2019) 675–685
https://doi.org/10.1016/j.giec.2019.06.007
1052-5157/19/© 2019 Elsevier Inc. All rights reserved.

giendo.theclinics.com

Large colorectal lesions are defined as equal to or greater than 20 mm (2 cm). With their larger size, it is more difficult to perform en bloc resection (removal in 1 piece or by 1 snare resection) and they often require piecemeal resection (PR). Or they may have a pathologic positive margin unless the lesion is a pedunculated polyp.[3] PR is a known risk factor for recurrence at the resection site and, therefore, it is necessary to perform surveillance colonoscopy at shorter intervals and to attempt further endoscopic treatment as required until complete eradication of dysplasia is achieved.[3,4] Past reports of recurrence with PR were high and surgical resection was often preferred for lesions when ER was considered likely technically impossible owing to the lesion size or configuration, or for those suspected to contain invasive cancer. Surgical resection can be performed by removing only the segment of colon containing the large polyp or lesion; however, the rates of morbidity and mortality associated with surgery are much higher than with endoscopic therapy. Recent improvement of techniques for ER and endoscopic treatment of complications, and (more notably) the emergence of a new technique called endoscopic submucosal dissection (ESD), has enabled endoscopists to perform ER on large colonic lesions much more effectively. Endoscopic treatment is now applied to a wider range of sizes and locations of colorectal lesions. The line between lesions for surgery and for ER has become obscure and, currently, nearly all benign polyps and some likely malignant lesions should be considered for ER regardless of size and location.

This article discusses the indications and limitations of each treatment modality. The goal is to guide readers when to consider ER (either endoscopic mucosal resection [EMR] or ESD) and surgery.

ENDOSCOPIC TREATMENT OF LARGE COLON POLYPS

ER is the least invasive treatment of colorectal polyps. Polypectomy is a common practice for endoscopists who perform colonoscopy or flexible sigmoidoscopy. Polypectomies are performed for lesions smaller than 10 mm, and fluid-assisted polypectomy or EMR are performed for lesions that are sessile or flat and larger than 10 mm. Lesions larger than 20 mm require proper techniques to complete resection during the initial attempt. Scarring may prevent complete eradication of a polyp or dysplasia, and surgical treatment can then become inevitable. Large colorectal lesions are usually defined as equal to or greater than 20 mm, for which resection in 1 piece becomes more challenging, often resulting in PR.

LARGE COLON POLYPS: LESION FACTOR

Colon polyps demonstrate various sizes and configurations, and the Paris classification is a useful tool to describe lesions.[5,6]

Paris classification type 0-Ip is a pedunculated polyp that is rather easily removed en bloc by the snare resection method, even when larger than 2 cm. If the snare can be passed over the polypoid portion (head), then resection can be performed at the stalk, leaving an adequate margin to provide meaningful information about possible invasion into the stalk for an assessment of the risk for metastasis (Haggitt criteria).[7]

Paris classification type 0-II is a superficial lesion, including flat elevated, flat, and depressed lesions (0-IIa, IIb, IIc). Of these, 0-IIa and 0-IIb lesions larger than 1 cm are usually called laterally spreading lesions or laterally spreading tumors (LSTs). A 0-IIc lesion is a depressed-type tumor that is considered to have a higher potential to contain high-grade dysplasia (HGD) or invasive cancer, even when small.[8-10]

Conventional polypectomy with a snare is typically difficult for large superficial (0-II) lesions, and EMR or saline-assisted polypectomy is essential to remove lesions effectively. As mentioned previously, EMR on large superficial lesions often result in PR (en bloc resection rate from 13% to 54% at advanced resection centers).[3,4,11,12] Well-planned EMR is essential to effectively eradicate large lesions because prior attempt of resection causes fibrosis, which can prevent or reduce adequate lifting for EMR and reduce the efficacy of endoscopic treatment at subsequent attempts if residual dysplasia remains or recurs.[10]

Paris classification type 0-Is is a sessile lesion. It is well known that the large nodule mixed within the 0-IIa type is called mixed-type LST; this type of lesion is best described as type 0-IIa+Is. Detailed investigations of histology showed that large (>10 mm) nodules are often associated with submucosally invasive cancer.[9,13] It was suggested that these nodules be first removed by EMR to preserve architecture for accurate pathologic analysis.

It is important to stratify colorectal lesions into high risk and low risk to contain HGD or invasive cancer because this is critical for choosing the method of resection. Some colorectal lesions contain and demonstrate signs of malignant transformation on the surface, but these signs are often subtle and are overlooked if examination is not carefully done. When malignant transformation is suspected, the depth of invasion should be evaluated endoscopically to exclude noncandidates for ER. High-resolution endoscopy and an advanced imaging study (eg, chromoendoscopy with or without magnification, optical chromoendoscopy) are extremely helpful to identification of the area and assessing the possibility of the presence of invasive cancer.[14,15] A report from Japan suggested that the risk factors of deeper invasion into submucosa include lesion with a large (≥10 mm) nodule, defined area of depression, loss of surface pit pattern, wall stiffness, prominent redness, convergence, and tumor size greater than or equal to 20 mm. However, only a large nodule within LST-granular type, wall stiffness, loss of surface pit pattern, and tumor size greater than or equal to 20 mm within LST-nongranular type were independent risk factors in a multivariate analysis.[9] Similar findings were reported in an Australian study, in which 0-IIa+IIc classification, nongranular type, and type V pit pattern (destructed or loss of surface pit pattern) were risk factors for submucosal invasive cancer.[10]

If ER is to be performed, the area of concern (for possible HGD or cancer) needs to be removed en bloc (ie, 1 piece) to assess the depth of pathologic invasion and margins, and to evaluate for oncological curative resection.

Curative resection is defined as margin-negative resection for dysplasia (low-grade and high-grade) combined with no to minimum risk for metastasis for tumor stage (T)-1 cancer. The presence of invasive cancer (invasion beyond muscularis mucosae into the submucosal layer) is classified as T1 by tumor-node-metastasis (TNM) classification and is considered as a risk factor for regional (lymph node metastasis) and distant metastasis.[16] Lymphovascular invasion (LVI), single-cell invasion (or tumor budding [TB]), and deep depth of invasion are considered to be high-risk indicators for metastasis. Cancer invasion depth less than 1000 μm is considered the cutoff for low risk for metastasis in the absence of other factors.[17] Surgical resection is recommended for patients with lesions with features of invasive cancer with high-risk factors (LVI and TB), and LVI has been demonstrated as the strongest indicator for regional metastasis.[18–20] Primary surgical treatment can be considered for a T1 lesion with a known risk for lymph node metastasis (LNM) of approximately 10%. However, endoscopic diagnosis lacks specificity for T1 disease and many patients may undergo surgical resection for adenoma or carcinoma in situ (Tis disease) with no risk for metastasis.

In addition, accumulating data suggest there is a low-risk category in T1 lesions. Low-risk T1 lesion for LNM is defined by 3 factors: (1) absence of a poorly differentiated component, (2) invasion depth less than 1000 μm (1 mm) or Haggitt level 1 to 3 for pedunculated polyp, and (3) no evidence of LVI and TB.[7,17,18,21–23] It is best to obtain proper pathologic evaluation on the tumor and to stratify the need for additional formal oncological surgical resection. High-quality EMR or ESD with proper postresection tissue processing provides a large section of undisrupted tissue for detailed pathologic review. A pinned specimen allows a proper cutting plane for pathologic evaluation for deep and lateral margins (**Fig. 1**). Small and partially resected and curled specimens without orientation make pathologic evaluation nearly impossible and may cause overstaging (eg, invasive cancer cannot be excluded). In this case, surgical resection is often recommended; however, most patients would be proven to have noninvasive disease after surgery. On the other hand, when there is a high degree of suspicion for a T1 lesion with deep submucosal invasion (>1000 μm) or higher T stage (T2–T4), primary surgical resection should be chosen to avoid unnecessary endoscopic intervention and associated complications.

ENDOSCOPIC RESECTION: ENDOSCOPIC MUCOSAL RESECTION VERSUS ENDOSCOPIC SUBMUCOSAL DISSECTION

ER is the mainstay of treating colorectal dysplasia. En bloc resection is ideal whenever possible, allowing proper pathologic evaluation with low recurrence rate. En bloc resection by EMR for large colorectal lesions, if successful, can achieve a low recurrence rate (2.3%–3%).[3,4,12] However, most ERs for large colorectal lesions result in PR (~70%), which is associated with a higher rate of residual or recurrent dysplasia than en bloc resection.[3,11,24,25] One study showed the recurrence rate was associated with the number of resection pieces at index EMR.[4] For noncancerous polyps or lesions, eradication by endoscopic piecemeal resection can be achieved with high efficacy because residual or recurrent adenoma can be treated by repeated endoscopic treatments. A high success rate (90%–93%) of eradication of residual adenoma by endoscopic retreatment during surveillance colonoscopy was reported by a systematic review and a large multicenter study from Australia.[12,24] On the other hand, large noncancerous and early cancerous lesions can also be treated effectively by ESD, with a high en bloc rate that results in very low risk for residual lesion and recurrence

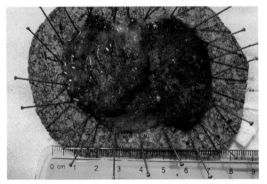

Fig. 1. Proper processing of resected specimen. The specimen was pinned onto the cork board with its cut surface on the bottom. Proper perpendicular sections in 2-mm intervals need to be performed after orienting specimen for detailed pathologic evaluation.

of dysplasia (0.9%–2%).[24,26,27] Complications are higher with ESD compared with EMR. Bleeding risk is 4.8% to 5.7% for ESD compared with 2.3% to 3.5% for EMR. Perforation risk is 4.8% to 5.7% compared with 0.9% to 1.4%, respectively.[11,27,28] However, most perforations are small and identified during the procedure and can be treated effectively with endoscopic treatment. Systematic reviews report surgery for complication was higher for ESD versus EMR (3% vs 0.4%), analyzing publications from 2009 to 2013.[11] More recent systematic reviews on ESD, from 2007 to 2016, showed lower surgery rates for adverse events (1.1%), especially in publications from Asia (0.8%). Other significant differences are a need for dedicated training for ESD and longer procedure times, which heavily depend on location, the presence of submucosal fibrosis and neoplastic vessels, the size of the lesion, and the operator's experience.[26] As experience accumulates and training and devices improve for ESD procedures, procedure time and the rate of complications are expected to be reduced.

SURGERY: LAPAROSCOPIC COLECTOMY AND TRANSANAL ENDOSCOPIC MICROSURGERY OR TRANSANAL MINIMALLY INVASIVE SURGERY

Colorectal surgery with appropriate lymphadenectomy is the standard of care for colorectal carcinoma, with appropriate neoadjuvant or adjuvant therapy decided on by a multidisciplinary team.[29–32] Controversy exists on the management of T1 disease. In Japanese guidelines in which low-risk criteria for T1 colorectal cancer is accepted, surveillance without surgery is suggested for low-risk T1 colorectal cancer. In Western countries, T1 cancer is usually not divided in subgroups and additional surgical resection is generally recommended. However, the benefit of additional surgical resection for all endoscopically resected T1 disease was questioned in some retrospective studies because there were no significant differences seen with additional surgery compared with clinical follow-up.[18,22,33] Recurrent disease was predictive when high-risk markers (LVI, poorly differentiated type, or positive resection margin) were present and selective surgery only for those high-risk group was suggested.

Surgery was reported to be performed on many benign colorectal lesions despite the advancement and availability of ERs.[34,35] Colon surgery poses fairly high comorbidity rates (16.4% overall and 14.7% for benign colonic neoplasms) and the cost is significantly higher than ER.[36]

For large rectal lesions or localized rectal cancers, transanal endoscopic microsurgery (TEM) has been an alternative to ER. Locally advanced rectal cancer needs proper multimodal therapy and highly invasive surgery (abdominoperineal resection); proper tumor staging is of utmost importance. For a proper pathologic assessment of the risks and need for adjuvant therapy, en bloc resection is recommended for all rectal lesions suspected to contain invasive cancer.[31] In the past, TEM was preferred over EMR for suspicious rectal lesions or large rectal lesions. In 2011, a decreased recurrence rate for large adenoma was reported, showing the benefit of TEM compared with piecemeal EMR.[37] However, this may not be true in the modern era of improved EMR technique (10%–20% residual adenoma rate compared with the published 31% rate). Adverse events with TEM were more severe than with EMR.

In the past decade, ESD started to offer a larger en bloc resection of rectal lesions, thus the value of ESD compared with TEM was explored. In a systematic review, publications on ESD between 2006 and 2010 were compared with those on TEM between 1996 and 2011. En bloc resection rates were 87.8% and 98.7% ($P<.001$) and margin negative resection (R0) rates were 74.6% and 88.5% ($P<.001$), respectively.[38]

Complications were similar but recurrence rates were 2.6% and 5.2% (*P*<.001), respectively. It is important to comment that these data are from the early phase of colorectal ESD (2006–2010) compared with established TEM data (most are from 2003–2011) and thus results were favorable for TEM. There have been improved outcomes of ESD over the last decade as experience accumulates and techniques and technologies have improved. More recent case series study initially showed a similar R0 resection rate of ESD compared with TEM (81.8% vs 84.6%, respectively) with similar recurrence rate (9% vs 15%, respectively).[39] The same group reported updated results from 2008 to 2017 in abstract form in 2019, showing an improved R0 resection rate of ESD (85%) compared with the rate of TEM (83%) and a statistically significant (*P* = .0001) lower recurrence rate of ESD (1.3%) compared with the rate of TEM (24.1%).[40]

As a new technique for resection of rectal lesions, transanal minimally invasive surgery (TAMIS) was reported in 2010 as an alternative to TEM.[41] This surgical platform uses ordinary laparoscopic instruments. TAMIS is gaining popularity with high-margin negative resection for local resection of dysplasia or low-risk early-stage cancer.[42,43] A clinical study comparing TAMIS to ESD for early rectal neoplasms is ongoing and outcomes are awaited.

PUTTING IT ALTOGETHER: WHICH TREATMENT FOR WHICH LESIONS?

Large colorectal lesions have a higher risk for containing invasive cancer than smaller lesions; however, the overall rate is low (7.8%).[24] If the lesion is only epithelial dysplasia (low-grade dysplasia and HGD), then eradication is the goal to prevent future risk for colorectal cancer, and piecemeal EMR may be more suitable and preferred for its cost and availability.

If the recurrence rate with multimodal piecemeal EMR is shown to be almost as low as ESD, it would be very difficult to argue for ESD rather than piecemeal EMR, provided that the diagnostic sensitivity for cancer within the polyp is adequately high and can prevent PR of invasive cancer. However, due to the limitation on the sensitivity, as well as the specificity, for diagnosing invasive cancer within the lesion, ESD provides benefit for patients who have a borderline or suspicious lesion for invasive cancer, and ESD would provide the complete surgical specimen to stratify the patients who would and would not benefit from additional surgery by the histologic high-risk criteria (see previous discussion of lesion factor and surgery).

Further argument can be made that the ESD procedure and techniques are evolving and ESD is becoming safer and easier, with shorter procedure time aided by new techniques and tools. With the advancement of ESD, reduction of time and complications would further complicate arguments on EMR versus ESD versus surgery. ESD may become the preferred method for many large colorectal lesions at experienced centers, with fewer complications and reduced procedure time. In particular, rectal lesions with a substantial risk of cancer are good candidates for ESD because the morbidity of adjuvant surgical procedures for endoscopically resected rectal cancers is greater than that for colonic cancers.

In the Australian Colonic EMR (ACE) study, invasive cancers were found in 43 lesions (4.3%) out of 1000 successfully resected specimens after excluding suspicious lesions for invasive cancers.[12] All subjects were referred for surgical resection. In a Japanese multicenter study comparing EMR and ESD, invasive cancers were found in 151 lesions (9.9%) out of 1524 lesions, but less than one-third of subjects were considered to be in high-risk group and they were referred to surgery. If all patients were treated with ESD and proper pathological information were obtained, are there patients who can be spared from having colorectal surgery? To address this question, Bahin and colleagues[44] performed an analysis of the cost-effectiveness of the application of wide-field (WF)-EMR or ESD for large colorectal lesions using current the Australian fee schedule. It was reported that the selective ESD application was the most cost-effective, preventing 19 additional surgeries per 1000 cases, when ESD was performed only when submucosally invasive cancer was suspected by the presence of 1 or more of: depressed configuration, disrupted surface pit pattern, and non-lifting sign. The comparison groups were WF-EMR and surgery for the high-risk group versus universal ESD. This calculation included the cost for initial procedures, hospital stays, treatments for adverse events calculated by assumed complication rates for all treatment modalities, surveillance colonoscopies, and additional treatments as expected by current recurrence rate. The ESD cost was calculated as similar to TEM done with anesthesia compared with moderate sedation in WF-EMR. Also, ESD included a 2-night hospital stay, increasing the overall cost. In the author's practice, ESD procedures are more frequently done on an outpatient basis and recent improvements of the ESD procedure reduced the procedure time and rates of complications. Surveillance colonoscopy interval is recommended to be lengthened to 12 months if margin-negative resection is achieved, reducing the cost for surveillance colonoscopy. The cost calculation would be much more favorable for ESD if those changes are taken into account.

ESD was suggested to have higher rate of additional surgery compared with EMR (ESD 6.9%–9.9% vs EMR 4.1%–5.8%).[11,27] This is likely due to the inclusion of larger lesions and high-risk lesions containing invasive cancers in the ESD group. In a systematic review, the ESD group contained twice as many submucosal cancers (8.5%) as the EMR group (4.8%).[27]

Large colorectal lesions that show any substantial chance of invasive cancer should undergo en bloc resection by a proper technique if feasible, most likely by ESD. Upfront ER should be chosen for lesions with HGD or suspected early-stage cancer with a technique to allow R0 resection. Multiple publications showed that initial ER of malignant lesion would not alter surgical outcomes if additional surgery is required.[20,45,46]

The European Society of Gastrointestinal Endoscopy, the American Society for Gastrointestinal Endoscopy, and the American Gastroenterological Association have published their assessment and guideline for ESD on colorectal lesions.[47–49] For rectal lesions, good-quality ESD offers comparable outcomes, with lower complication rates, cost, and recurrence rates than TEM. Although it is expected that ESD will offer a lower cost option, further data are awaited to compare the benefits of TAMIS and ESD for large risky lesions.

SUMMARY

For large colorectal lesions with no clear signs of deeply invasive cancer, ER (EMR or ESD) should be the gold standard. High-quality WF-EMR is highly effective. ESD offers the benefits of lower recurrence rates, preserved histology for risk stratification for lesions suspected to contain cancer, and overall reduced costs when applied to selected lesions. If HGD or invasive cancer is suspected, ESD is a better ER method if available. Lesion selection for ESD is expected to expand when ESD becomes less time-consuming with lower adverse event rates and more expert ESD centers are available. Primary surgery should be the gold standard for suspected deep submucosal cancers, as well as more advanced tumor stages (**Fig. 2**).

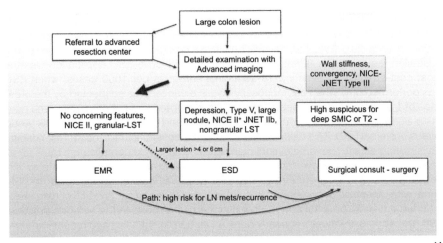

Fig. 2. Proposed algorithm of a treatment selection for large colorectal lesions using NICE[14] and JNET[15] classifications. LN met, lymph node metastasis; JNET, Japan NBI Expert Team; NICE, Narrow-Band Imaging International Colorectal Endoscopic; SMIC, submucosally invasive cancer.

REFERENCES

1. Jayanna M, Burgess NG, Singh R, et al. Cost analysis of endoscopic mucosal resection vs surgery for large laterally spreading colorectal lesions. Clin Gastroenterol Hepatol 2016;14(2):271–8.e1-2.

2. Law R, Das A, Gregory D, et al. Endoscopic resection is cost-effective compared with laparoscopic resection in the management of complex colon polyps: an economic analysis. Gastrointest Endosc 2016;83(6):1248–57.

3. Belderbos TD, Leenders M, Moons LM, et al. Local recurrence after endoscopic mucosal resection of nonpedunculated colorectal lesions: systematic review and meta-analysis. Endoscopy 2014;46(5):388–402.

4. Oka S, Tanaka S, Saito Y, et al. Local recurrence after endoscopic resection for large colorectal neoplasia: a multicenter prospective study in Japan. Am J Gastroenterol 2015;110(5):697–707.

5. The Paris endoscopic classification of superficial neoplastic lesions: esophagus, stomach, and colon: November 30 to December 1, 2002. Gastrointest Endosc 2003;58(6 Suppl):S3–43.

6. Endoscopic Classification Review Group. Update on the paris classification of superficial neoplastic lesions in the digestive tract. Endoscopy 2005;37(6):570–8.

7. Haggitt RC, Glotzbach RE, Soffer EE, et al. Prognostic factors in colorectal carcinomas arising in adenomas: implications for lesions removed by endoscopic polypectomy. Gastroenterology 1985;89(2):328–36.

8. Kudo S, Kashida H, Tamura T. Early colorectal cancer: flat or depressed type. J Gastroenterol Hepatol 2000;15(Suppl):D66–70.

9. Uraoka T, Saito Y, Matsuda T, et al. Endoscopic indications for endoscopic mucosal resection of laterally spreading tumours in the colorectum. Gut 2006; 55(11):1592–7.

10. Moss A, Bourke MJ, Williams SJ, et al. Endoscopic mucosal resection outcomes and prediction of submucosal cancer from advanced colonic mucosal neoplasia. Gastroenterology 2011;140(7):1909–18.

11. Arezzo A, Passera R, Marchese N, et al. Systematic review and meta-analysis of endoscopic submucosal dissection vs endoscopic mucosal resection for colorectal lesions. United European Gastroenterol J 2016;4(1):18–29.

12. Moss A, Williams SJ, Hourigan LF, et al. Long-term adenoma recurrence following wide-field endoscopic mucosal resection (WF-EMR) for advanced colonic mucosal neoplasia is infrequent: results and risk factors in 1000 cases from the Australian Colonic EMR (ACE) study. Gut 2015;64(1):57–65.

13. Saito Y, Fujii T, Kondo H, et al. Endoscopic treatment for laterally spreading tumors in the colon. Endoscopy 2001;33(8):682–6.

14. Hayashi N, Tanaka S, Hewett DG, et al. Endoscopic prediction of deep submucosal invasive carcinoma: validation of the narrow-band imaging international colorectal endoscopic (NICE) classification. Gastrointest Endosc 2013;78(4):625–32.

15. Sano Y, Tanaka S, Kudo SE, et al. Narrow-band imaging (NBI) magnifying endoscopic classification of colorectal tumors proposed by the Japan NBI expert team. Dig Endosc 2016;28(5):526–33.

16. Weiser MR. AJCC 8th edition: colorectal cancer. Ann Surg Oncol 2018;25(6): 1454–5.

17. Kitajima K, Fujimori T, Fujii S, et al. Correlations between lymph node metastasis and depth of submucosal invasion in submucosal invasive colorectal carcinoma: a Japanese collaborative study. J Gastroenterol 2004;39(6):534–43.

18. Meining A, von Delius S, Eames TM, et al. Risk factors for unfavorable outcomes after endoscopic removal of submucosal invasive colorectal tumors. Clin Gastroenterol Hepatol 2011;9(7):590–4.

19. Nascimbeni R, Burgart LJ, Nivatvongs S, et al. Risk of lymph node metastasis in T1 carcinoma of the colon and rectum. Dis Colon Rectum 2002;45(2):200–6.

20. Nozawa H, Ishihara S, Fujishiro M, et al. Outcome of salvage surgery for colorectal cancer initially treated by upfront endoscopic therapy. Surgery 2016; 159(3):713–20.

21. Kobayashi H, Higuchi T, Uetake H, et al. Resection with en bloc removal of regional lymph node after endoscopic resection for T1 colorectal cancer. Ann Surg Oncol 2012;19(13):4161–7.

22. Ikematsu H, Yoda Y, Matsuda T, et al. Long-term outcomes after resection for submucosal invasive colorectal cancers. Gastroenterology 2013;144(3):551–9 [quiz: e514].

23. Backes Y, Elias SG, Groen JN, et al. Histologic factors associated with need for surgery in patients with pedunculated T1 colorectal carcinomas. Gastroenterology 2018;154(6):1647–59.

24. Hassan C, Repici A, Sharma P, et al. Efficacy and safety of endoscopic resection of large colorectal polyps: a systematic review and meta-analysis. Gut 2016; 65(5):806–20.

25. Emmanuel A, Lapa C, Ghosh A, et al. Risk factors for early and late adenoma recurrence after advanced colorectal endoscopic resection at an expert Western center. Gastrointest Endosc 2019;90(1):127–36.

26. Fuccio L, Hassan C, Ponchon T, et al. Clinical outcomes after endoscopic submucosal dissection for colorectal neoplasia: a systematic review and meta-analysis. Gastrointest Endosc 2017;86(1):74–86 e17.

27. Fujiya M, Tanaka K, Dokoshi T, et al. Efficacy and adverse events of EMR and endoscopic submucosal dissection for the treatment of colon neoplasms: a meta-analysis of studies comparing EMR and endoscopic submucosal dissection. Gastrointest Endosc 2015;81(3):583–95.

28. De Ceglie A, Hassan C, Mangiavillano B, et al. Endoscopic mucosal resection and endoscopic submucosal dissection for colorectal lesions: a systematic review. Crit Rev Oncol Hematol 2016;104:138–55.
29. Vogel JD, Eskicioglu C, Weiser MR, et al. The American Society of colon and rectal surgeons clinical practice guidelines for the treatment of colon cancer. Dis Colon Rectum 2017;60(10):999–1017.
30. Labianca R, Nordlinger B, Beretta GD, et al. Early colon cancer: ESMO clinical practice guidelines for diagnosis, treatment and follow-up. Ann Oncol 2013; 24(Suppl 6):vi64–72.
31. Glynne-Jones R, Wyrwicz L, Tiret E, et al. Rectal cancer: ESMO clinical practice guidelines for diagnosis, treatment and follow-up. Ann Oncol 2017;28(suppl_4): iv22–40.
32. Hashiguchi Y, Muro K, Saito Y, et al. Japanese Society for Cancer of the Colon and Rectum (JSCCR) guidelines 2019 for the treatment of colorectal cancer. Int J Clin Oncol 2019. [Epub ahead of print].
33. Belderbos TD, van Erning FN, de Hingh IH, et al. Long-term recurrence-free survival after standard endoscopic resection versus surgical resection of submucosal invasive colorectal cancer: a population-based Study. Clin Gastroenterol Hepatol 2017;15(3):403–11.e1.
34. van Nimwegen LJ, Moons LMG, Geesing JMJ, et al. Extent of unnecessary surgery for benign rectal polyps in the Netherlands. Gastrointest Endosc 2018; 87(2):562–70.e1.
35. Peery AF, Cools KS, Strassle PD, et al. Increasing rates of surgery for patients with nonmalignant colorectal polyps in the United States. Gastroenterology 2018;154(5):1352–60.e3.
36. Zogg CK, Najjar P, Diaz AJ, et al. Rethinking priorities: cost of complications after elective colectomy. Ann Surg 2016;264(2):312–22.
37. Barendse RM, van den Broek FJ, Dekker E, et al. Systematic review of endoscopic mucosal resection versus transanal endoscopic microsurgery for large rectal adenomas. Endoscopy 2011;43(11):941–9.
38. Arezzo A, Passera R, Saito Y, et al. Systematic review and meta-analysis of endoscopic submucosal dissection versus transanal endoscopic microsurgery for large noninvasive rectal lesion s. Surg Endosc 2014;28(2):427–38.
39. Kawaguti FS, Nahas CS, Marques CF, et al. Endoscopic submucosal dissection versus transanal endoscopic microsurgery for the treatment of early rectal cancer. Surg Endosc 2014;28(4):1173–9.
40. Kawaguti FS, Kimura CMS, Marques CF, et al. Endoscopic submucosal dissection (ESD) versus transanal endoscopic microsurgery (TEM) for the treatment of early rectal cancer: comparison of long term outcomes. Gastrointest Endosc 2019;89(6):AB406.
41. Atallah SB, Albert MR. Transanal minimally invasive surgery (TAMIS) versus transanal endoscopic microsurgery (TEM): is one better than the other? Surg Endosc 2013;27(12):4750–1.
42. Martin-Perez B, Andrade-Ribeiro GD, Hunter L, et al. A systematic review of transanal minimally invasive surgery (TAMIS) from 2010 to 2013. Tech Coloproctol 2014;18(9):775–88.
43. deBeche-Adams T, Hassan I, Haggerty S, et al. Transanal Minimally Invasive Surgery (TAMIS): a clinical spotlight review. Surg Endosc 2017;31(10):3791–800.
44. Bahin FF, Heitman SJ, Rasouli KN, et al. Wide-field endoscopic mucosal resection versus endoscopic submucosal dissection for laterally spreading colorectal lesions: a cost-effectiveness analysis. Gut 2018;67(11):1965–73.

45. Rickert A, Aliyev R, Belle S, et al. Oncologic colorectal resection after endoscopic treatment of malignant polyps: does endoscopy have an adverse effect on onco-logic and surgical outcomes? Gastrointest Endosc 2014;79(6):951–60.
46. Lopez A, Bouvier AM, Jooste V, et al. Outcomes following polypectomy for malig-nant colorectal polyps are similar to those following surgery in the general pop-ulation. Gut 2019;68(1):111–7.
47. Pimentel-Nunes P, Dinis-Ribeiro M, Ponchon T, et al. Endoscopic submucosal dissection: European Society of Gastrointestinal Endoscopy (ESGE) Guideline. Endoscopy 2015;47(9):829–54.
48. Committee AT, Maple JT, Abu Dayyeh BK, et al. Endoscopic submucosal dissec-tion. Gastrointest Endosc 2015;81(6):1311–25.
49. Draganov PV, Wang AY, Othman MO, et al. AGA Institute clinical practice update: endoscopic submucosal dissection in the United States. Clin Gastroenterol Hep-atol 2019;17(1):16–25 e11.

Lesion Retrieval, Specimen Handling, and Endoscopic Marking in Colonoscopy

Arshish Dua, MD[a], Brian Liem, DO[b], Neil Gupta, MD, MPH[c],*

KEYWORDS

- Polyp retrieval • Retrieval device • Specimen integrity • Pathology
- Endoscopic marking • Tattoo

KEY POINTS

- Retrieval of resected lesions is critical for pathologic analysis in endoscopic polypectomy. Various techniques and devices can be used for retrieval.
- Pathologic analysis requires appropriate lesion handling and preparation. For large polyps undergoing en bloc resection, pinning and marking of lesions after resection is frequently indicated.
- Endoscopic marking or endoscopic tattooing guides future surgical localization and endoscopic surveillance. Tattoo mediums and techniques have been well described.

 Video content accompanies this article at http://www.giendo.theclinics.com.

INTRODUCTION

Endoscopic polypectomy within the colon with successful polyp retrieval is essential to the process of reducing colorectal malignancy–associated mortality.[1] The population-based benefit from colonoscopic polypectomy arises from the significant reduction in colorectal cancer incidence.[2] Successful retrieval specifically enables the histopathologic analysis of polyp tissue, which helps determine subsequent management, complete eradication, and endoscopic surveillance interval.[3,4] The US Multi-Society Task Force on Colorectal Cancer previously recommended that endoscopists be able to retrieve at least 95% of polyps for histopathologic analysis, with the European Society

---

Disclosure Statement: No relevant financial or nonfinancial relationships to disclose.
[a] Division of Gastroenterology, Loyola University Medical Center, Stritch School of Medicine, 2160 South 1st Avenue, Building 54, Room 167, Maywood, IL 60153, USA; [b] Gastroenterology Fellowship, Division of Gastroenterology, Stritch School of Medicine, Loyola University Medical Center, 2160 South 1st Avenue, Building 54, Room 167, Maywood, IL 60153, USA; [c] Digestive Health Program, Division of Gastroenterology, Stritch School of Medicine, Loyola University Medical Center, 2160 South 1st Avenue, Building 54, Room 167, Maywood, IL 60153, USA
* Corresponding author.
E-mail address: negupta@lumc.edu

Gastrointest Endoscopy Clin N Am 29 (2019) 687–703
https://doi.org/10.1016/j.giec.2019.06.002
1052-5157/19/© 2019 Elsevier Inc. All rights reserved.

of Gastrointestinal Endoscopy recommending a similar benchmark.[5,6] Specimen processing and endoscopic marking are additional critical components of lesion management. Current emphasis on quality indicators in endoscopy invariably influences the need to successfully retrieve polyp tissue. Adenoma detection rate cannot be definitively determined at this time without histopathologic analysis of tissue.

LESION RETREIVAL

Retrieval of lesions additionally allows for assessment of tissue margins and complete eradication, which may further aid in management and surveillance decisions. Some evidence supports the occurrence of interval colorectal cancer at sites of incompletely resected adenomatous tissue.[7] Histopathologic analysis is not without cost; "resect and discard" or "diagnosis and disregard" strategies have been proposed for diminutive polyps 1 to 5 mm in size that undergo thorough endoscopic vetting and documentation with added visualization technologies such as narrow band imaging.[8] The requirement of validated endoscopic visualization approaches, expert experience, and high confidence in assessment when using these techniques is recommended by both the American Society for Gastrointestinal Endoscopy and the European Society of Gastrointestinal Endoscopy.[9,10] Further potential situations to forego polyp retrieval involve polypectomy in known polyposis syndromes where eradication of small or very flat polyps may be of more importance than pathologic analysis. Despite validated alternate approaches to polyp analysis, polyp retrieval with subsequent histopathology remains the gold-standard technique for definitive polyp analysis and can be applied to polyps of all sizes and appearances if amendable to endoscopic removal.

Polyp retrieval failure rates have been reported from 2% to 16.5%, with more recent studies reporting success rates greater than 90%.[11–14] Previous data have shown that polyps less than 5 mm in diameter, polyps in right side of the colon, resection via cold snare, and inadequate bowel preparation are contributing factors for retrieval failure.[14,15] Numerous devices are used to retrieve polyps, including forceps, snares with or without suction techniques, pronged graspers, baskets, and retrieval nets[16] (**Fig. 1, Table 1**). Few randomized controlled trials exist comparing specific retrieval methods, and approaches are largely dictated by polyp size and removal method.[16,17]

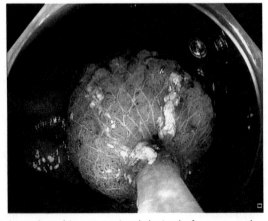

Fig. 1. Resected lesion gripped in net retrieval device before removal.

Table 1
Retrieval devices with advantages and disadvantages

Retrieval Devices	Advantages	Disadvantages
Forceps	• Ease of use • Cost • Low retrieval failure rate • Ability to continue endoscopic examination without withdrawal	• Highly limited capacity • Potential incomplete resection • Potential maceration of tissue
Snares	• Larger capacity size • Single-use device for intervention and retrieval • Ability to continue endoscopic examination (periodic dropping of lesion)	• Limited capacity (one large polyp) • Cost of additional device • Potential architectural tissue destruction (cutting into pieces) • Potential loss of polyp • May require complete withdrawal of endoscope
Graspers	• Larger capacity size	• Cost of additional device • Potential maceration and loss of polyp • Better options with similar capacity • Generally requires removal of endoscope
Baskets	• Larger capacity size • Ability to collect multiple pieces	• Cost of additional device • Potential maceration and loss of polyp pieces • Generally requires removal of endoscope
Retrieval Nets	• Largest capacity size • Maintains polyp integrity • Ease of use in collecting multiple pieces without loss	• Cost of additional device • Generally requires removal of endoscope

RESECTION TECHNIQUES AFFECTING RETRIEVAL

Biopsy forceps removal of polyps obviates a simple retrieval process via pulling of the closed forceps device containing the intact resected polyp out of the corresponding insertion channel. Various jaw configurations and sizes are commercially available for use with or without needle-spike designs, which aid in deeper tissue sampling as well as multiple tissue collections in a single pass.[18] Hot biopsy forceps have largely been abandoned due to increased risks of use without demonstrated added benefits when compared with cold techniques.[18] Biopsy forceps retrieval is limited to diminutive polyps generally 1–3 mm in size if polyp integrity is to be maintained with clear margins.[18,19] The advantages of this method are continuance of endoscopic examination and intervention without withdrawal as well as excellent retrieval rates, as the polyp is embedded within the jaws/spike of the forceps and is unlikely to be lost in the instrument channel on withdrawal. Randomized controlled trials and systematic reviews have however demonstrated that small and diminutive polyp integrity may be compromised with use of standardized forceps versus jumbo or cold snare techniques.[20,21] In addition, incomplete resection is another concern that has been demonstrated in quickly repeated endoscopic studies following initial forceps removal of polyp.[22,23] Hence forceps retrieval use is limited to 1 to 3 mm polyps and care should be taken to ensure that the entire polyp is removed. A potential approach to determine if the polyp can be resected and retrieved in one piece with clear margins using biopsy forceps is by comparing the closed forceps size with adjacent polyp size; if the closed forceps seem larger in diameter than the polyp, complete retrieval in one piece may be more successful.

Cold snaring is especially useful for removal of polyps up to 9 mm in size and potentially limits complication rates from alternative techniques such as hot snare cautery. It is more frequently being used for polyp removal, as recent randomized controlled trials as well as meta-analyses have shown cold snaring to be a more efficient and equally efficacious modality for removal of polyps less than 10 mm when compared with hot snare cautery.[24,25] Cold snaring has however been associated with increased failure in polyp retrieval, although some studies have demonstrated retrieval rates as high as 98%.[14,15,26] During cold excision tenting of the polyp after snare closure is not necessary or recommended, as injury to deeper tissues is very unlikely. Lack of tenting will enable the polyp to remain in place after cutting, thereby facilitating suction or other removal directly at the polypectomy site. If tenting is used the polyp has the potential to rapidly propel in the direction of the tented force and can hinder the retrieval process, as the polyp may not remain at its original location.[27] This contrasts with hot snaring technique, as tenting and slight decompression of the lumen to thicken the colonic walls is recommended to avoid complications of thermal injury. An additional technique for polyp retrieval during cold snaring is to pull the snared polyp into the suction channel before transection[26] This technique negates the need for suction or other retrieval within the colonic lumen because the polyp will already be inside the given channel and can be used for polyps located in difficult locations such as the upper left endoscopic field. A potential disadvantage of this technique includes the inability to visualize the polyp during transection and potential maceration of the polyp.

RETRIEVAL AND SPECIFIC DEVICES

After a polyp is removed via snare techniques with or without piecemeal excision and if the polyp or its corresponding fragments remain in the colonic lumen, retrieval can be accomplished by various methods depending on size and device used[16,18,19] (see **Table 1**). If the polyp or fragments of polyp can move through the instrument channel, which is generally 2.8 to 3.7 mm in size, they can be placed in the 5 o'clock position in the endoscopic field of view and suctioned into the endoscope through the shaft and umbilical apparatus into a corresponding collection device.[17] Polyps larger than the channel size can be suctioned through the endoscope as well with deformation and conformation within the channel. An attached trap or other end retrieval device facilitates collection when suctioning through the entire endoscope is used.

Various devices used for end collection include simple gauze or mesh placed between the suction nipple and tubing, an independent plastic compartment with a removable filter, or a multicompartment device that can be rotated to collect individual specimens[17,28] (**Table 2**). Polyps or fragments that get stuck typically in the umbilicus

Table 2 Collection devices on retrieval		
Collection Devices	**Advantages**	**Disadvantages**
Simple gauze or mesh placed between the suction nipple and tubing	• Lack of device • Low cost	• Loss of polyp during collection • Potential maceration
Independent plastic compartment with a removable filter	• Ease of collection	• Increased cost of device • Assistant management
Multicompartment device that can be rotated	• Ease of collection • Ability to collect multiple samples in one device	• Increased cost of device • Requires stepwise collection with rotation • Assistant management

of the endoscope can be evacuated with use of additional water or saline suctioning. Sources of fluid include water from an incorporated instrument jet or residual fluid in the colonic lumen. An alternative approach particularly when neither is available includes the use of a syringe filled with water or saline that can be injected into the instrument port with simultaneous suctioning applied facilitating clearance of the polyp. If a polyp cannot be found after suctioning retrieval attempts, effort should be made to inspect the biopsy channel port, the suction trumpet apparatus, and the suction aperture for potential distally occluded polyp.[17]

Further variations on suction removal exist, including using placement of a finger over the aperture of the removed suction valve with or without filterable material for direct polyp retrieval at the aperture and/or increased suction power. Suctioning removal techniques for polyps too large to fit through the instrument channel include applied continuous suction with the resected lesion gripped flush with the distal channel aperture and subsequent removal of the entire endoscope. This technique has the disadvantage of potentially obscuring the endoscopic view, and tissue can easily be dislodged along tight corners and narrow lumen or lost if the polyp is subsequently suctioned into the instrument channel.[29] Another "channel occlusion" technique eliminates need of trap devices whereby a snare or catheter occludes the instrument channel except for the distal end and the polyp is suctioned into the distal tip of the endoscope with proximal occlusion from the catheter or snare.[29] Removal of the endoscope is again required with subsequent pushing out of the resected polyp with the snare or catheter from the distal instrument channel. Advantages include ability to maintain endoscopic view, but further intervention with retrieval again cannot be accomplished in one insertion, as endoscope removal is required to collect the initial lesion. Polyp integrity via fragmentation or distortion may be a disadvantage of channel suctioning techniques in general particularly of larger polyps not amendable to inherent channel size. The clear advantage of polyp suction through instrument channel regardless of end retrieval method is the ability to continue the endoscopic examination and further needed interventions without withdrawal of the endoscope. Obvious cost benefits exist as well as novel retrieval devices would not be needed.

For lesions too large to be suctioned through the instrument channel, alternative retrieval devices such as snares, multipronged forceps, baskets, and nets can be used[16,18,19] (see **Table 1**). A variety of snare options are commercially available with sizes up to 30 to 40 mm, costs ranging from 16 to 615 USD, and reusability options.[16,19] A single large excised polyp can be retrieved using the snare by maintaining a firm grasp on the polyp and pulling out the endoscope with the snare several centimeters ahead in view as the polyp follows to maintain endoscopic visualization. The polyp should be pulled snug to the colonoscope tip when exiting the rectum. One distinct advantage of using the snare for retrieval is that the large polyp can be periodically dropped and other lesions identified, excised, and potentially retrieved without removing the endoscope. A disadvantage is that one insertion retrieval is limited to one large polyp or one large polyp with fragments or additional lesions that can be retrieved via suction or forceps biopsy. In addition, risk of polyp transection with the gripped snare and dislodgement of the polyp itself is possible particularly when pulling through tight spots on removal with the endoscope.

Graspers are commercially available in 2 to 5 prong designs with sizes up to 25 mm, have costs ranging from 52 to 694 USD, and contain reusability options.[16] As an advantage they can be used to retrieve single polyps generally 10 to 15 mm in size. However, insufficient grasping strength, potential architectural destruction of polyp tissue, and alternative methods for retrieval (with the similar disadvantage of requiring removal of the endoscope) exist, which limit their use in everyday practice specifically for polyp retrieval. A similar removal could be accomplished with snare grip as well without adding the cost of an additional device.

If there are multiple large pieces after piecemeal polypectomy and/or multiple large polyps from the same colonic section, a basket or mesh retrieval device can be used (**Fig. 2**). Baskets are commercially available in 4 to 6 wire configurations with accommodating sizes generally up to 30 mm in diameter and cost 52 to 327 USD, have reusable options, and generally can be used to retrieve polyps or pieces of polyp up to 20 mm in size.[16] An advantage of baskets as well as net retrieval devices is the ability to pick up multiple polyps or pieces of polyp in one endoscopic insertion. The device can be reopened and closed to collect as many polyps or pieces of polyp that the basket can accommodate. With baskets the space between the wires limits the size of polyp that can be retrieved. The technique of gently pressing the forward tip of the basket against the colonic lumen may allow for further opening of the wires to accommodate tissue. Disadvantages include requirement of endoscope removal, dislodgement of previously recovered tissue when new pieces are collected, additional device cost, and capacity limitations.

Retrieval nets are commercially available from several manufacturers. They offer maximum diameters of 30 mm and come in various configurations. Multiple pieces of polyp or multiple polyps can be retrieved with these devices in a similar repetitive opening and closing manner as basket devices with maintenance of polyp integrity[30] (Video 1). This retrieval is accomplished by positioning the excised lesion at the 6 o' clock location, opening of the retrieval net on top of the tissue, placing the concave aspect of the net over the lesion, and subsequently closing the device (**Fig. 3**). Polyps and pieces of any size can be collected in this manner with repeated opening and snug closure of the mesh, which will push large fragments to the distal end of the retrieval device, facilitating pick up of further large pieces. Ease of collection, lack of dislodgement of previously collected pieces, and polyp integrity seem to be additional advantages to these devices. The disadvantage of not being able to remove further lesions until the endoscope is removed remains.

Often polyps that have been excised migrate from the polypectomy site out of endoscopic view and may be difficult to find and retrieve. Using direction and flow of a water stream jet administered at the polypectomy site can aid in retrieval.[11,31] If the jet of

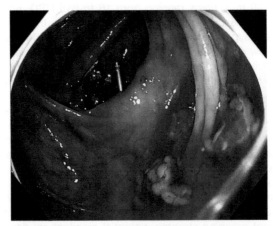

Fig. 2. Polypectomy pieces collected in the first distal pool after piecemeal excision in an endoscopic mucosal resection procedure. Retrieval of all pieces in one insertion can be accomplished using net or basket devices if capacity permits.

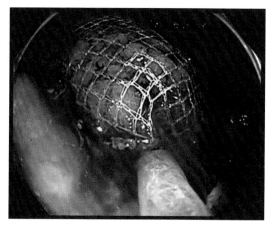

Fig. 3. Concave aspect of laying net device on top of resected lesion with the net partially closed.

water flows forward away from the site, attempts at suctioning or exploring the first proximal pool of fluid should be attempted. If the water jet obscures the field of view flowing in a downward or backward direction, the first distal pool should similarly be explored for polyp retrieval (see **Fig. 2**). An additional method for retrieval uses cutting of large polyps or sections of polyp into smaller pieces, which are subsequently removed via suction technique. The clear disadvantage of this approach is potential disruption of histopathologic analysis of polyp tissue and loss of fragmented polyp sections. In cases of suspected cancerous lesions and lesions removed with en bloc resection, the polyp should be removed in one piece. Resected pedunculated polyps should always be removed intact and without fragmentation. Increased accuracy of the pathologic analysis particularly of lateral and deep margins for tumor involvement is attained with en bloc resection. The advantage of the cut in pieces approach is that it avoids the need for reintubation for reexamination and intervention, as polyps can be continually removed in one insertion session.

SPECIMEN PROCESSING

Appropriate lesion handling after polypectomy and polyp retrieval is critical to successful histopathologic analysis. Multidisciplinary interaction and communication with pathologists aids in tissue collection and analysis.[32,33] Communication may help elucidate amount of fixative solution needed, jar capacity, and recommended specimen orientations.[34] Effort should be made to remove all polyp tissue for pathologic assessment in one endoscopic evaluation to limit repeat endoscopy, exposure to sedation, and cost.

POLYP INTEGRITY

Maintaining polyp integrity at the time of polypectomy contributes to lower recurrence rates and incidence of residual lesions and aids in determining suitability for future oncologic resection.[33,35] Furthermore, en bloc resection of polyps is recommended when technically feasible, as it facilitates better lesion retrieval, integrity, and pathologic analysis.[35,36] No distinct size cutoff value for one-piece polypectomy has been recommended. It is reasonable to attempt removal in one piece for nonpedunculated lesions up to 2 cm in size with conventional techniques and/or endoscopic mucosal resection. Further en bloc resection for lesions larger than 2 cm can be accomplished with advanced techniques such as endoscopic submucosal dissection.[34–36] In piecemeal polypectomy, residual polyp tissue should be removed via snare, and for flat lesions that cannot be gripped via avulsion with forceps. If concern exists toward cancerous features of a polyp, it is important when lifting to inject adjacent to the polyp rather than through the polyp to maintain integrity for pathologic analysis (Video 2). Incomplete eradication of polyp tissue and polyp recurrence is correlated with significant piecemeal resection, increased use of thermal ablation, and large polyp size.[35] Pedunculated lesions should be removed en bloc by transection through the stalk regardless of size.

LESION HANDLING

Resected lesions and their sites can be examined for potential complications when clinical suspicion or procedure complexity warrants (**Fig. 4**). A "target sign" or pale white to gray focal area on a resection site may indicate muscularis propria partial or full-thickness transection and increases concern for perforation.[37] Immediately after polyp resection and retrieval the specimen should be gently submerged into a jar containing fixation fluid for architectural preservation and desiccation minimization. Pinning and/or inking of margins before fixation is recommended for large en bloc resections particularly when cancerous features are appreciated. Ten percent buffered formalin solution is typically used, as it provides exceptional fixation and allows for optimal routine histologic staining.[34] Individual jar submission with detailed specimen labeling is generally recommended. Polyps resected from different locations should be submitted in separate containers; generally accepted locations that are also reported in pathologic analysis include the cecum, right (ascending) colon, hepatic flexure, transverse colon, splenic flexure, left (descending) colon, sigmoid colon, and rectum.[38] Multiple small or diminutive polyps with similar and benign endoscopic features from the same colonic location can potentially be submitted in one specimen jar to reduce collection times, materials, and cost. The European guidelines for quality assurance in pathology in colorectal cancer screening and surveillance however recommend that each resected lesion be placed in a separate container.[39,40] Lesion shape should be noted on the pathology request, so that the pathologist or technician will be alert to the stalk of pedunculated lesions.

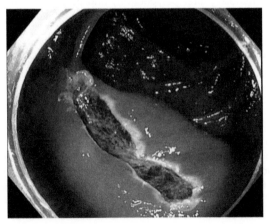

Fig. 4. Inspection of endoscopic mucosal resection site with lack of concerning features.

Mucosal excision margins can be better assessed by inking or placing pins at the margins of the specimen with the mucosal surface facing upwards.[40] This is particularly important in en bloc endoscopic mucosal resection and endoscopic submucosal dissection specimens, as assessment of lateral and deep margins may be obscured with formalin fixation alone.[40] Lateral and deep margin assessment is advantageous to confirming curative nature of resection; a margin of 1 mm or greater is used as one component of curative declaration in en bloc resection analysis of lesions.[40–42] For large pedunculated polyps optimal positioning includes cauterization and cutting approximately one-third down the stalk from the polyp head. This increases the chance that the polyp will have clear margins when submitted for pathologic analysis while balancing the need to mitigate postpolypectomy complications such as bleeding and perforation. With very large pedunculated polyps that necessitate piecemeal removal, it is crucial to send the base of the polyp adjacent to or nearest to the stalk in a separate jar to the pathologist, as this piece of tissue is the most important to analyze for cancerous change. In piecemeal polypectomy it is recommended to embed the entire submitted lesion to exclude invasive malignancy.[40] The use of endoscopic submucosal dissection offers excellent pathologic analysis as well as complete eradication of the given lesion in one session due to the en bloc nature of the resection.[41] The need for appropriate pathologic analysis is weighed against the increased complication rate of perforation, bleeding, and need for hospitalization in these procedures. Endoscopic mucosal resection offers a quicker and safer means of removal of large sessile lesions; however, pathologic analysis is often hindered by the piecemeal resection of these polyps and the recurrence rate is higher possibly due to residual polyp at the site between piecemealed sections.[42]

ENDOSCOPIC TATTOOING

Endoscopic marking (or endoscopic "tattoo" placement) for future localization of colonic lesions has been used since 1975.[43] Tattooing should be used for sites that may require future operative intervention or endoscopic surveillance of the resection site. With regard to endoscopic surveillance, polyps that require piecemeal resection and/or large polyps that are endoscopically resected should be marked with some exceptions depending on lesion location. The increased prevalence of laparoscopic colorectal intervention makes prior endoscopic marking of significant importance, as identification of lesions with palpation and direct inspection is limited.[44] As many as 14% of lesion locations identified during endoscopic evaluation can be inaccurate when compared with subsequent surgical identification.[45] Studies have additionally reported localization issues after endoscopic evaluation, including wrong segment removal, blind removal, and inability to identify lesions necessitating laparotomy.[46–49]

Various techniques including clipping and radiologic approaches to preoperative lesion marking and endoscopic surveillance have been used, with endoscopic tattooing remaining the gold standard for lesion marking.[47,50,51] A systematic review of 38 nonrandomized and observational studies analyzing tumor localization errors in patients undergoing surgical colorectal cancer resection found a pooled incidence of localization errors with conventional colonoscopy of 15.4% compared with 9.5% when using endoscopic tattooing (mean difference 5.9%, confidence interval .65–11.14, $P = .03$).[51] Tattooing may increase the quality of lymph node analysis at the time of colorectal cancer resection as well.[52] The American Society for Gastrointestinal Endoscopy and the European Society of Gastrointestinal Endoscopy have endorsed the use of endoscopic tattooing for suspicious lesions after or without endoscopic polypectomy for future endoscopic surveillance and/or surgical localization.[53–55]

Although no formal guideline recommendations are available on specifics of endoscopic tattooing pertaining to size, endoscopic appearance, placement, or tattoo mediums, various approaches have been well described, which aid future colorectal lesion management and surveillance.[53,54]

WHAT TO INJECT

Multiple staining dyes, including India ink, Carbon black, methylene blue, indigo carmine, indocyanine green, toluidine blue, isosulfan blue, and hematoxylin/eosin, have been tested or used in endoscopic tattooing[53,56–60] (**Table 3**). Of these only indocyanine green, India ink, and carbon black persist in tissue greater than 48 hours, limiting use of other agents for this purpose.[16,19] Although India ink has been shown to persist in tissue years after injection, indocyanine green seems limited in time span, with one study showing precipitous drops in visible marking at surgery 8 days or greater from tattoo placement.[58,61]

A sterile, prediluted suspension containing fine purified carbon particles was developed named SPOT (GI supply, Camp Hill, Pennsylvania) and is the only Food and Drug Administration–approved medium available specifically for endoscopic tattooing.[59] SPOT persists in tissue for years and additionally lacks potential mucosal irritants including ethylene glycol, phenols, ammonia, or shellacs that are found in India ink preparations.[57,59,62] It furthermore does not require sterilization or tedious dilution, making it easy for clinical use.[53,59,63] However, the cost and availability of SPOT solution in comparison with India ink may limit its use in endoscopic tattooing. Both India ink when used in a 1:100 dilution with avoidance of stronger concentrations and SPOT preparations have excellent safety profiles and efficacy, with studies demonstrating none or rare complications most of which include clinically silent peritoneal spillage or mild peritonitis.[56,57,59,64,65] Their long-term staining qualities make them the preferred tattooing mediums for future endoscopic surveillance and surgical localization[53] (see **Table 3**). Idiopathic inflammatory bowel disease, tumor inoculation, abscess, remote extraintestinal staining, hematoma, and inflammatory pseudotumor have been rarely reported as potential serious

Table 3
Dye mediums and long-term persistence in colonic tissue

Dye Medium	Persists in Tissue >48 hrs	Persists in Tissues >8 d	Potential to Persist in Tissue for Years	Recommended in Tattooing
Pure carbon black	+	+	+	+ (gold standard, FDA approved)
India ink	+	+	+	+ (cheaper, 1:100 dilution or more preferred)
Indocyanine green	+	−	−	−
Methylene blue	−	−	−	−
Indigo carmine	−	−	−	−
Toluidine blue	−	−	−	−
Isosulfan blue	−	−	−	−
Hematoxylin/ eosin	−	−	−	−

Abbreviation: FDA, Food and Drug Administration.

adverse effects with SPOT and India ink preparations in dilutions stronger than 1:100.[65,66]

SUBMUCOSAL INJECTION

Targeted submucosal injection of dye is critical with most complications of invisible lesion, diffuse bowel wall staining, and peritoneal spillage likely a consequence of shallow, deep, or transmural administration of dye medium[56,57,65] (**Fig. 5**). Needle insertion depth of 8 mm is enough to penetrate colonic wall. However, oblique insertion at a 45-degree angle to a limited depth of 5 mm confines injection to the submucosal space[67] (**Fig. 6**). Inserting 2 to 4 mm of needle tip into the colonic mucosa in tangential fashion and then slightly lifting to observe the needle impression within the submucosal space is a reasonable approach to targeted submucosal administration. The needle should be inserted at this oblique angle to avoid penetration of deeper colonic layers. On injecting in the submucosa, immediate engorgement should be appreciated or the injection stopped. Aliquots of 0.5 to 1.0 mL can be administered at each injection site[53] (Video 3).

Various saline test injection techniques have been described to identify the submucosal plane before dye injection with India ink and/or SPOT.[64,68–70] One method includes initial saline injection into the submucosal space with replacement of the saline syringe with a syringe containing dye in a one-time needle insertion approach.[64,68] An alternative includes creation of a saline bleb with needle withdrawal and second needle insertion into the submucosal bleb with subsequent injection from a syringe filled with dye medium.[69,70] These techniques may increase effectiveness of subsequent operative identification, reduce complications of intraperitoneal spillage, and result in more precise tattoo placements although randomized controlled trial data are lacking.[68,69]

QUADRANT MARKING

The European Society of Gastrointestinal Endoscopy recommends tattooing sites of piecemeal polypectomy, endoscopic mucosal resection, endoscopic submucosal dissection, difficult to detect polyps, and proven or suspected malignant lesions.[71]

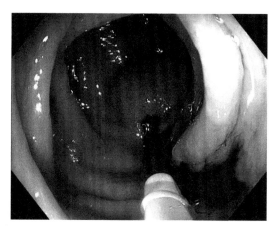

Fig. 5. Inking performed at the distal site of a concerning lesion. The intraluminal spillage appreciated in this picture at the end of injection should be avoided by instillation of 0.5 to 1.0 mL aliquots only and immediately stopping injection when seen.

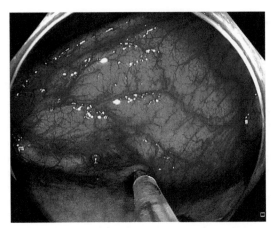

Fig. 6. Initial submucosal needle insertion immediately before injecting tattoo dye after endoscopic mucosal resection of a lesion. Note the oblique angle of insertion and slight tenting to identify needle impression.

Tattooing approach and placement in various scenarios have not been standardized or compared in randomized controlled trials.[56,72] There has been a call for guideline standardization of endoscopic tattooing for complication prevention and for successful surgical localization or endoscopic surveillance.[72]

When marking the location of suspected cancerous lesion for surgical resection, the 3 to 4 quadrant approach has emerged as the preferred method for endoscopic marking.[51,56,73] One or two quadrant tattoos may be inadequate for surgical localization, as they can be hidden by pericolonic fat, mesentery, omentum, or the posterior abdominal wall at the time of surgical evaluation.[73] Orientation within the colonic lumen is difficult to discern and targeting of the antimesenteric region to prevent this issue is subsequently hindered. Dye aliquots of 0.5 to 1.0 mL can be injected with conventional or saline bleb technique in a 4-quadrant, circumferential manner, 2 to 3 cm distal from the given site. Tattooing the distal edge of a lesion in this 4-quadrant manner can be helpful to the surgeon, as it aids in identifying the extent of distal dissection needed for a given operative procedure. This is particularly helpful with left-sided distal lesions with or without rectal involvement. Often lesions located in the right side of the colon or cecum and the rectum do not require marking, as these locations can be easily and reliably identified endoscopically. Precise description of tattoo location in relationship to a lesion or polypectomy site should be included in the operative report. Terminology should specify tattoo orientation to the lesions using words such as "opposite to" or "3 cm distal and immediately to the left of" of the lesion. Accompanying photo documentation is essential in guiding future identification as well as surgical and endoscopic management (Video 4).

If marking for purposes of endoscopic surveillance, tattooing should ideally occur after polypectomy is complete, as injection marking into the surrounding submucosa can cause rolling of tissue into the polypectomy defect obscuring visualization and further removal of residual polyp. Tattooing the proximal or distal aspect of a polypectomy site can aid in endoscopic surveillance and is generally adequate for this purpose with only 1 to 2 distinct injections at a given site needed. Whether the distal, proximal, or both ends of the site are marked should be noted. If tattooing is administered on only one side of the polypectomy site, ensuring appropriate documentation of which side was tattooed in the endoscopic report is necessary.

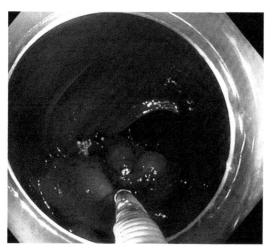

Fig. 7. Injection of dye medium underneath and immediately adjacent to a lesion. This should be avoided to prevent future difficulty in locating the lesion as well as complications at the time of resection.

Every effort should be made to avoid direct inoculation of the lesion/site and instead the endoscopist should target areas 2 to 3 cm away from a given lesion/site (see Video 3). Avoidance of direct lesion injection mitigates scarring, which may increase risk for future perforation particularly during subsequent endoscopic removal[74] (**Fig. 7**). It may also limit future endoscopic visualization of polyp invasion or potential needle track seeding of tumor.

PHOTO AND OTHER DOCUMENTATION

Descriptive wording as well as measurement of lesion location, specifics of tattooing approach, and photo documentation should be detailed in all endoscopic reports[53,56] (**Box 1**). A method includes documentation of gross location, lesion location in centimeter from the anal verge, tattoo method, and subsequent photo documentation pre- as well as post-tattoo placement. With the increased use of endoscopic tattooing multiple prior marked sites emerge as a confusion issue in subsequent surgical localization and endoscopic intervention or surveillance.[56] All old markings at the time of

---

Box 1
Appropriate documentation in endoscopic tattooing

Components of Tattoo Documentation
  Specify location in colon
  Specify distance from anal verge
  Specify amount of tattoos placed (generally 4 for surgical referral, 1–2 for endoscopic referral)
  Specify tattoo locations in terms of proximal centimeter, distal centimeter, or both proximal and distal centimeter to lesion site and/or polypectomy location
  Specify orientation in relationship to lesion (opposite wall, same wall, detailed description)
  Specify relevant colonic landmarks when tattooing deferred
  Provide thorough visual documentation (photo and video when feasible)
  Provide thorough documentation of all the abovementioned in endoscopic reports

endoscopic evaluation should be described and measured in the same manner as new tattoos. Lack of standardized guidelines make photo and descriptive documentation of tattooing crucial, as approaches vary among providers. If further accuracy in tattooing location is sought scope guide or radiographic techniques can be used to further localize the site of marking although these techniques are seldom used for this purpose.

SUMMARY

Lesion retrieval, specimen processing, and endoscopic marking are essential components to successful colorectal polypectomy and contribute to the process of reducing colorectal cancer incidence as well as mortality. Mastery of these techniques is recommended for any successful clinical endoscopist.

SUPPLEMENTARY DATA

Supplementary data related to this article can be found online at https://doi.org/10.1016/j.giec.2019.06.002.

REFERENCES

1. Zauber AG, Winawer SJ, O'brien MJ, et al. Colonoscopic polypectomy and long-term prevention of colorectal-cancer deaths. N Engl J Med 2012;366(8):687–96.
2. Winawer SJ, Zauber AG, Ho MN, et al. Prevention of colorectal cancer by colonoscopic polypectomy. The National Polyp Study Workgroup. N Engl J Med 1993;329(27):1977–81.
3. Rex DK, Boland CR, Dominitz JA, et al. Colorectal cancer screening: recommendations for physicians and patients from the U.S. Multi-Society task force on colorectal cancer. Am J Gastroenterol 2017;112(7):1016–30.
4. Lieberman DA, Rex DK, Winawer SJ, et al. Guidelines for colonoscopy surveillance after screening and polypectomy: a consensus update by the US Multi-Society task force on colorectal cancer. Gastroenterology 2012;143(3):844–57.
5. Rex DK, Bond JH, Winawer S, et al. Quality in the technical performance of colonoscopy and the continuous quality improvement process for colonoscopy: recommendations of the U.S. Multi-Society task force on colorectal cancer. Am J Gastroenterol 2002;97(6):1296–308.
6. Kaminski MF, Thomas-gibson S, Bugajski M, et al. Performance measures for lower gastrointestinal endoscopy: a European Society of Gastrointestinal Endoscopy (ESGE) quality improvement initiative. Endoscopy 2017;49(4):378–97.
7. Pabby A, Schoen RE, Weissfeld JL, et al. Analysis of colorectal cancer occurrence during surveillance colonoscopy in the dietary polyp prevention trial. Gastrointest Endosc 2005;61(3):385–91.
8. Hewett DG, Rex DK. Colonoscopy and diminutive polyps: hot or cold biopsy or snare? Do I send to pathology? Clin Gastroenterol Hepatol 2011;9(2):102–5.
9. Abu dayyeh BK, Thosani N, Konda V, et al. ASGE Technology Committee systematic review and meta-analysis assessing the ASGE PIVI thresholds for adopting real-time endoscopic assessment of the histology of diminutive colorectal polyps. Gastrointest Endosc 2015;81(3):502.e1–16.
10. Kamiński MF, Hassan C, Bisschops R, et al. Advanced imaging for detection and differentiation of colorectal neoplasia: European Society of Gastrointestinal Endoscopy (ESGE) guideline. Endoscopy 2014;46(5):435–49.

11. Waye JD, Lewis BS, Atchison MA, et al. The lost polyp: a guide to retrieval during colonoscopy. Int J Colorectal Dis 1988;3(4):229–31.
12. Nakao NL. Combined cautery and retrieval snares for gastrointestinal polypectomy. Gastrointest Endosc 1996;44(5):602–5.
13. Webb WA, Mcdaniel L, Jones L. Experience with 1000 colonoscopic polypectomies. Ann Surg 1985;201(5):626–32.
14. Fernandes C, Pinho R, Ribeiro I, et al. Risk factors for polyp retrieval failure in colonoscopy. United European Gastroenterol J 2015;3(4):387–92.
15. Komeda Y, Suzuki N, Sarah M, et al. Factors associated with failed polyp retrieval at screening colonoscopy. Gastrointest Endosc 2013;77(3):395–400.
16. Diehl DL, Adler DG, Conway JD, et al. Endoscopic retrieval devices. Gastrointest Endosc 2009;69(6):997–1003.
17. Waye J. It ain't over 'til it's over: retrieval of polyps after colonoscopic polypectomy. Gastrointest Endosc 2005;62(2):257–9.
18. Barkun A, Liu J, Carpenter S, et al. Update on endoscopic tissue sampling devices. Gastrointest Endosc 2006;63(6):741–5.
19. Carpenter S, Petersen BT, Chuttani R, et al. Polypectomy devices. Gastrointest Endosc 2007;65(6):741–9.
20. Draganov PV, Chang MN, Alkhasawneh A, et al. Randomized, controlled trial of standard, large-capacity versus jumbo biopsy forceps for polypectomy of small, sessile, colorectal polyps. Gastrointest Endosc 2012;75(1):118–26.
21. Raad D, Tripathi P, Cooper G, et al. Role of the cold biopsy technique in diminutive and small colonic polyp removal: a systematic review and meta-analysis. Gastrointest Endosc 2016;83(3):508–15.
22. Woods A, Sanowski RA, Wadas DD, et al. Eradication of diminutive polyps: a prospective evaluation of bipolar coagulation versus conventional biopsy removal. Gastrointest Endosc 1989;35(6):536–40.
23. Peluso F, Goldner F. Follow-up of hot biopsy forceps treatment of diminutive colonic polyps. Gastrointest Endosc 1991;37(6):604–6.
24. Fujiya M, Sato H, Ueno N, et al. Efficacy and adverse events of cold vs hot polypectomy: a meta-analysis. World J Gastroenterol 2016;22(23):5436–44.
25. Kawamura T, Takeuchi Y, Asai S, et al. A comparison of the resection rate for cold and hot snare polypectomy for 4-9 mm colorectal polyps: a multicentre randomised controlled trial (CRESCENT study). Gut 2018;67(11):1950–7.
26. Deenadayalu VP, Rex DK. Colon polyp retrieval after cold snaring. Gastrointest Endosc 2005;62(2):253–6.
27. Hewett DG. Cold snare polypectomy: optimizing technique and technology (with videos). Gastrointest Endosc 2015;82(4):693–6.
28. Sano Y, Kaihara T, Ito H, et al. A novel endoscopic device for retrieval of polyps resected from the colon and rectum. Gastrointest Endosc 2004;59(6):716–9.
29. Chey WD. The channel occlusion technique: a novel method of retrieving polyps following snare resection. Am J Gastroenterol 2000;95(6):1608–9.
30. Miller K, Waye JD. Polyp retrieval after colonoscopic polypectomy: use of the Roth Retrieval Net. Gastrointest Endosc 2001;54(4):505–7.
31. Waye JD. Techniques of polypectomy: hot biopsy forceps and snare polypectomy. Am J Gastroenterol 1987;82(7):615–8.
32. Weinstein WM. Mucosal biopsy techniques and interaction with the pathologist. Gastrointest Endosc Clin N Am 2000;10(4):555–72, v.
33. Fukami N. Large colorectal lesions: is it possible to stratify the lesions for optimal treatment in the right hands? Gastrointest Endosc 2016;83(5):963–5.

34. Sharaf RN, Shergill AK, Odze RD, et al. Endoscopic mucosal tissue sampling. Gastrointest Endosc 2013;78(2):216–24.
35. Belderbos TD, Leenders M, Moons LM, et al. Local recurrence after endoscopic mucosal resection of nonpedunculated colorectal lesions: systematic review and meta-analysis. Endoscopy 2014;46(5):388–402.
36. Oka S, Tanaka S, Saito Y, et al. Local recurrence after endoscopic resection for large colorectal neoplasia: a multicenter prospective study in Japan. Am J Gastroenterol 2015;110(5):697–707.
37. Swan MP, Bourke MJ, Moss A, et al. The target sign: an endoscopic marker for the resection of the muscularis propria and potential perforation during colonic endoscopic mucosal resection. Gastrointest Endosc 2011;73(1):79–85.
38. Washington MK, Berlin J, Branton P, et al. Protocol for the examination of specimens from patients with primary carcinoma of the colon and rectum. Arch Pathol Lab Med 2009;133(10):1539–51.
39. Von karsa L, Patnick J, Segnan N, et al. European guidelines for quality assurance in colorectal cancer screening and diagnosis: overview and introduction to the full supplement publication. Endoscopy 2013;45(1):51–9.
40. Quirke P, Risio M, Lambert R, et al. European guidelines for quality assurance in colorectal cancer screening and diagnosis. First Edition–Quality assurance in pathology in colorectal cancer screening and diagnosis. Endoscopy 2012; 44(Suppl 3):SE116–30.
41. Saito Y, Fukuzawa M, Matsuda T, et al. Clinical outcome of endoscopic submucosal dissection versus endoscopic mucosal resection of large colorectal tumors as determined by curative resection. Surg Endosc 2010;24(2):343–52.
42. Tanaka S, Kashida H, Saito Y, et al. JGES guidelines for colorectal endoscopic submucosal dissection/endoscopic mucosal resection. Dig Endosc 2015;27(4): 417–34.
43. Ponsky JL, King JF. Endoscopic marking of colonic lesions. Gastrointest Endosc 1975;22(1):42.
44. Holzman MD, Eubanks S. Laparoscopic colectomy. Prospects and problems. Gastrointest Endosc Clin N Am 1997;7(3):525–39.
45. Vignati P, Welch JP, Cohen JL. Endoscopic localization of colon cancers. Surg Endosc 1994;8(9):1085–7.
46. Yeung JM, Maxwell-armstrong C, Acheson AG. Colonic tattooing in laparoscopic surgery - making the mark? Colorectal Dis 2009;11(5):527–30.
47. Cho YB, Lee WY, Yun HR, et al. Tumor localization for laparoscopic colorectal surgery. World J Surg 2007;31(7):1491–5.
48. Wexner SD, Cohen SM, Ulrich A, et al. Laparoscopic colorectal surgery–are we being honest with our patients? Dis Colon Rectum 1995;38(7):723–7.
49. Frager DH, Frager JD, Wolf EL, et al. Problems in the colonoscopic localization of tumors: continued value of the barium enema. Gastrointest Radiol 1987;12(4): 343–6.
50. Ellis KK, Fennerty MB. Marking and identifying colon lesions. Tattoos, clips, and radiology in imaging the colon. Gastrointest Endosc Clin N Am 1997;7(3):401–11.
51. Acuna SA, Elmi M, Shah PS, et al. Preoperative localization of colorectal cancer: a systematic review and meta-analysis. Surg Endosc 2017;31(6):2366–79.
52. Dawson K, Wiebusch A, Thirlby RC. Preoperative tattooing and improved lymph node retrieval rates from colectomy specimens in patients with colorectal cancers. Arch Surg 2010;145(9):826–30.
53. Kethu SR, Banerjee S, Desilets D, et al. Endoscopic tattooing. Gastrointest Endosc 2010;72(4):681–5.

54. Fisher DA, Shergill AK, Early DS, et al. Role of endoscopy in the staging and management of colorectal cancer. Gastrointest Endosc 2013;78(1):8–12.
55. Zerey M, Hawver LM, Awad Z, et al. SAGES evidence-based guidelines for the laparoscopic resection of curable colon and rectal cancer. Surg Endosc 2013; 27(1):1–10.
56. Asgeirsson T. The need for standardization of colonoscopic tattooing of colonic lesions. Dis Colon Rectum 2015;58(2):268–9.
57. Nizam R, Siddiqi N, Landas SK, et al. Colonic tattooing with India ink: benefits, risks, and alternatives. Am J Gastroenterol 1996;91(9):1804–8.
58. Hammond DC, Lane FR, Welk RA, et al. Endoscopic tattooing of the colon. An experimental study. Am Surg 1989;55(7):457–61.
59. Askin MP, Waye JD, Fiedler L, et al. Tattoo of colonic neoplasms in 113 patients with a new sterile carbon compound. Gastrointest Endosc 2002;56(3):339–42.
60. Miyoshi N, Ohue M, Noura S, et al. Surgical usefulness of indocyanine green as an alternative to India ink for endoscopic marking. Surg Endosc 2009;23(2): 347–51.
61. Hammond DC, Lane FR, Mackeigan JM, et al. Endoscopic tattooing of the colon: clinical experience. Am Surg 1993;59(3):205–10.
62. Shatz BA, Weinstock LB, Swanson PE, et al. Long-term safety of India ink tattoos in the colon. Gastrointest Endosc 1997;45(2):153–6.
63. Salomon P, Berner JS, Waye JD. Endoscopic India ink injection: a method for preparation, sterilization, and administration. Gastrointest Endosc 1993;39(6):803–5.
64. Park JW, Sohn DK, Hong CW, et al. The usefulness of preoperative colonoscopic tattooing using a saline test injection method with prepackaged sterile India ink for localization in laparoscopic colorectal surgery. Surg Endosc 2008;22(2):501–5.
65. Trakarnsanga A, Akaraviputh T. Endoscopic tattooing of colorectal lesions: is it a risk-free procedure? World J Gastrointest Endosc 2011;3(12):256–60.
66. Cappell MS, Courtney JT, Amin M. Black macular patches on parietal peritoneum and other extraintestinal sites from intraperitoneal spillage and spread of India ink from preoperative endoscopic tattooing: an endoscopic, surgical, gross pathologic, and microscopic study. Dig Dis Sci 2010;55(9):2599–605.
67. Botoman VA, Pietro M, Thirlby RC. Localization of colonic lesions with endoscopic tattoo. Dis Colon Rectum 1994;37(8):775–6.
68. Fu KI, Fujii T, Kato S, et al. A new endoscopic tattooing technique for identifying the location of colonic lesions during laparoscopic surgery: a comparison with the conventional technique. Endoscopy 2001;33(8):687–91.
69. Sawaki A, Nakamura T, Suzuki T, et al. A two-step method for marking polypectomy sites in the colon and rectum. Gastrointest Endosc 2003;57(6):735–7.
70. Raju GS. What is new in tattooing? Custom tattooing. Gastrointest Endosc 2004; 59(2):328–9.
71. Ferlitsch M, Moss A, Hassan C, et al. Colorectal polypectomy and endoscopic mucosal resection (EMR): European Society of Gastrointestinal Endoscopy (ESGE) clinical guideline. Endoscopy 2017;49(3):270–97.
72. Moss A, Bourke MJ, Pathmanathan N. Safety of colonic tattoo with sterile carbon particle suspension: a proposed guideline with illustrative cases. Gastrointest Endosc 2011;74(1):214–8.
73. Hyman N, Waye JD. Endoscopic four quadrant tattoo for the identification of colonic lesions at surgery. Gastrointest Endosc 1991;37(1):56–8.
74. Ono S, Fujishiro M, Goto O, et al. Endoscopic submucosal dissection for colonic laterally spreading tumors is difficult after target tattooing. Gastrointest Endosc 2009;69(3 Pt 2):763–6.

Closure of Defects and Management of Complications

Gottumukkala Subba Raju, MD

KEYWORDS

- Colonoscopy • Endoscopic mucosal resection • Endoscopic submucosal dissection
- Perforation • Closure • Clips • Suturing device

KEY POINTS

- Several clip and suture devices are available for endoscopic hemostasis and perforation closure.
- These devices provide an opportunity to manage benign tumors of the colon without surgery.
- Most perforations after endoscopic mucosal resection are small and can be managed by through-the-scope clips without leaving the operating field.
- Prophylactic clip application for deep mural defects involving the muscularis propria without perforation prevents delayed perforations.

INTRODUCTION

During the last 2 decades, we have made substantial progress in colonoscopic screening procedures as well as implementation of endoscopic mucosal resection (EMR) and endoscopic submucosal dissection to prevent cancer and avoid surgery. However, the widespread acceptance of these therapeutic programs will not be possible without parallel implementation of safety measures to prevent and treat colonoscopic perforations. This article focuses on the colonoscopic closure of resection defects and perforations and the management of colon perforations.

HISTORY

Endoscopic closure of gastrointestinal tract perforations, whether by clips or sutures, has revolutionized endoluminal surgery. It allows us to close perforations immediately, thereby eliminating the need for surgery and the morbidity and mortality associated with it. It is interesting to note that before any detailed experimental studies were done to understand the role of endoscopic closure, clips were used to close perforations in patients. Professor Nib Soehendra's first successful closure of a gastric perforation after endoscopic resection of a leiomyoma in the 1990s opened up the field of

Disclosure Statement: No conflicts of interest.
Department of Gastroenterology, Hepatology & Nutrition, The University of Texas MD Anderson Cancer Center, Unit 1466, 1515 Holcombe Boulevard, Houston, TX 77030, USA
E-mail address: gsraju@mdanderson.org

endoscopic surgery.[1] A few years later, Hiroaki Yoshikane and his colleagues[2] reported the first successful repair of a colon EMR perforation with clips and Mana and his colleagues[3] reported the first successful closures of a sigmoid colon perforation from a mechanical injury. These studies provided impetus for subsequent animal studies to explore the application of endoluminal closure devices in the management of colonoscopic perforations.

EXPERIMENTAL STUDIES

Experimental studies on endoluminal closure of colonoscopic perforation using a porcine model using through-the-scope clips (TTSC), over-the-scope clips (OTSC), and suturing devices are summarized here (**Fig. 1**).

Through-the-scope-clips closure
- *Healing of perforation:* TTSC closure of a 1.5- to 2.0-cm linear colonoscopic perforation results in healing of perforation and prevents peritonitis.[4,5]
- *Leak-proof sealing of perforation:* TTSC closure can achieve a leak-proof sealing of both linear and circular colon perforations.[6,7]
- *Less peritoneal adhesions:* Endoluminal TTSC closure results in less peritoneal adhesions compared with surgical closure in a randomized, controlled porcine survival study, given the fact surgery requires damage to the peritoneum to reach the perforation site for closure.[8]
- *Limitation of TTSC closure:* Gaping perforations with sloping edges that are technically challenging for TTSC closure can be closed by endoluminal suturing devices.[9]

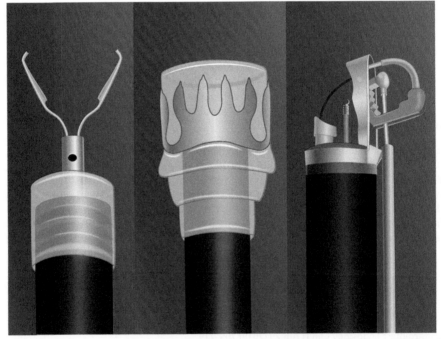

Fig. 1. Endoscopic closure devices for perforation closure. (*Left to right*) TTSC, OTSC, and over-the-scope-suturing devices. (© *2019 Gottumukkala Subba Raju.*)

Over-the-scope clips closure
- *Comparable secure closure:* TTSC and OTSC produce results comparable to hand-sewn colotomy closure in an ex vivo porcine colon model.[10]
- *Full-thickness resection closure:* Pilot studies demonstrated successful closure of defect after full-thickness resection.[11]

Suture closure
- *Closure of colon perforations:* Over-the-scope suturing device allows successful closure and healing of colonoscopic perforations in live porcine models.[12,13]
- *Closure of gaping wide perforations:* Through-the-scope suture closure allows successful closure of gaping wide perforations that cannot be closed by TTSCs.[9]
- *Closure of full-thickness resection:* A through-the-scope suture closure is successful in the closure of full-thickness resection defects of the colon.[12]

ENDOLUMINAL CLOSURE TOOLS
Closure Devices

A number of devices are currently available in the market to close defects (see **Fig. 1**).

A. Clips delivered through the endoscope (TTSC)
   a. Quick Clip (Olympus America Inc, Center Valley, PA)
   b. Resolution Clip (Boston Scientific Inc, Natick, MA)
   c. Instinct Clip (Cook Medical Inc, Bloomington, IN)
   d. Hemostatic clip (Changzhou JIUHONG Medical Instrument Co., Ltd. Changzhou, Jiangsu, China)
   e. Sureclip (Microtek Endoscopy, Ann Arbor, MI)
   f. Duraclip (ConMed, Utica, NY)
B. OTSC
   a. OTSC system (Ovesco Endoscopy AG, Tübingen, Germany)
   b. Padlock clip defect closure system (US Endoscopy, Mentor, OH)
C. Over-the-scope suturing device
   a. Overstitch Endoscopic Suturing System (Apollo Endosurgery, Austin, TX)

ENDOLUMINAL CLOSURE TECHNIQUES

Endoscopists benefit from mastering the use of one or more of the endoluminal closure techniques (**Fig. 2**).

Pros and cons of endoluminal closure devices
- TTSC can be used immediately after recognition of perforation to close the defect because they can be deployed through the endoscope without leaving the operating field.
- OTSC and over-the-scope suturing devices can close defects larger than those that can be closed by the TTSCs. However, both devices require removal of the endoscope from the perforation site to load the device on to the end of the endoscope and then reinsertion of the endoscope, followed by closure of the perforation.

Through-the-Scope Clip Closure
Principles for through-the-scope clip closure

- *Prompt closure:* Avoid spillage of colon contents by closing the perforation promptly with clips. This process may require keeping a couple of clips ready (out of their packets), especially during high-risk resections.

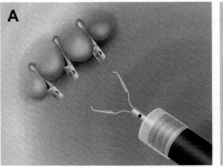
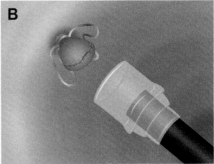
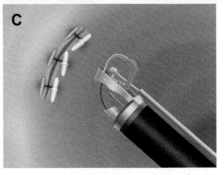

Fig. 2. Types of endoscopic closure. (*A*) TTSC closure of a perforation. (*B*) OTSC closure of a perforation. (*C*) Over-the-scope suture closure of a perforation. (© 2019 Gottumukkala Subba Raju.)

- *Maneuver clip–endoscope as a single unit* by keeping the clip close to the end of the endoscope; this offers technical advantage for successful closure.
- *Practice putting a cap for high-risk cases.* The routine use of a cap will allow the endoscopist to deflect the clips and facilitate endoscope passage to reach the defect to close it. In addition, because the current clips have a reopening function, one could negotiate through an area crowded by prior clips with the clip in the closed position and then apply it.
- *First clip application slightly away from the edge* allows to tent the edges of the perforation that permits deeper approximation of the edges with subsequent clip applications.
- *Apply clips at close quarters* to create a leak proof sealing.
- *Note: Clips retract on closure:* Gently push the clip during closure of the clip blades to compensate for the backward retraction of the blades as they close. This maneuver can be accomplished by either gently pushing the endoscope or clip catheter forward while slowly closing the clip (**Figs. 3** and **4**).
- *Aim for deep approximation of the edges of perforation with clip closure.* This is documented by the absence of any visible space between the blades of the clips, which is critical for a leak proof sealing.
- *Compensate for a loose approximation of the edges* (loose clip as evidenced by obvious space between the blades of the clip) by applying additional clips on either side of that clip to achieve deep approximation of the edges of perforation.
- *Extensive photodocument clip closure on both sides of the closure.* Both front side and back side, because sometimes the clip may slip and hang on just one edge. Take multiple photos.

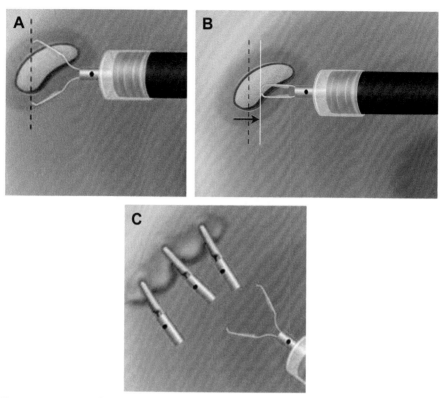

Fig. 3. TTSCs retract during closure resulting in superficial closure (*A–C*). (© *2019 Gottumukkala Subba Raju.*)

- *Decompress the colon after clip closure of the perforation.* The colon can get easily disrupted by the bowel distention required for colon examination; avoid the temptation of examining the rest of the colon. In addition, while gas escape through a free perforation does not generally increase the risk of infection, gas insufflation should be limited during repair to prevent mechanical complications from distention, including abdominal compartment syndrome and tension pneumothorax. The abdomen should be monitored for distention during repair of free perforation.

Basic clip closure techniques

a. *Transverse perforation closure:* Once the clip is opened, rotate the blades to align them perpendicular to the defect and engage the lower blade to the lower edge of a transverse perforation. Then, gently push the clip–endoscope unit while applying gentle suction to collapse the lumen so that the opposite edge of the perforation can be grasped as deeply as possible while the clip is slowly closed.

b. *Longitudinal perforation closure:* Start at the top end of the perforation and apply the clip just above the upper end of a longitudinal perforation to pucker the edges below for easier application of subsequent clips. Clips are placed from the top down to close longitudinal perforations starting away from the endoscope and working toward the endoscope or left to right for closure of circular or transverse perforations.

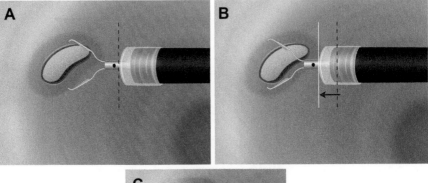

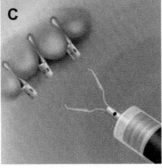

Fig. 4. Compensate clip retraction during closure either by pushing the endoscope or the clip for a deep approximation of the defect with clips (*A–C*). (© *2019 Gottumukkala Subba Raju.*)

Advanced clip closure techniques

Advanced clip closure techniques use additional devices to facilitate clip closure of larger perforations (**Fig. 5**).[14] A dual channel therapeutic endoscope is usually needed.

a. *Hold-and-drag closure technique using repositionable clips.* By grasping and dragging the anal edge to the oral side with a clip, both edges can approach each other. The defect is finally closed by reopening and placing the clip.

b. *Closure technique with small mucosal incisions to anchor the clip.* The defect is closed with hemoclips by hooking the small incisions and dragging the mucosal layer from one side to the other.

c. *Endoloop + TTSC (King closure).* An endoloop is delivered through 1 channel of endoscope. TTSCs are used to clip the endoloop to the defect circumferentially, followed by tightening of the endoloop to close the defect.[15]

d. *Eight-ring in combination with hemoclips.* After placement of the first clip with an 8-ring, the second clip hooking the 8-ring is placed on the contralateral edge.

e. *Clip-assisted closure using a foreign body forceps.* A large foreign body forceps is passed through one channel of the therapeutic scope and the edges of the defect are approximated followed by use of a TTSC through the other channel to close the defect.

f. *String clip suturing method.* The mucosal edges are approximated by pulling the string, which is anchored to both edges with hemoclips.

g. *Omental patch closure method.* The omentum is visualized through the perforation site and then suctioned into the gastric lumen before being grasped by the endoclips and securing it to the gastric mucosa or colonic mucosa thus creating an

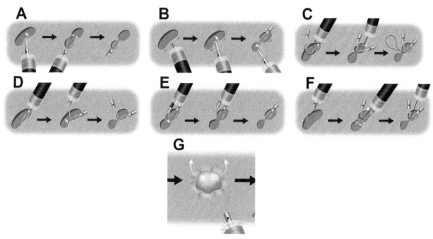

Fig. 5. Advanced techniques for TTSC closure. (*A*) Hold and drag technique. (*B*) Clip closure using small incisions to anchor the clip. (*C*) Endoloop-assisted clip closure. (*D*) An 8-ring assisted clip closure. (*E*) Foreign body forceps-assisted clip closure. (*F*) String suture-assisted clip closure. (*G*) Omental patch-assisted clip closure. (© *2019 Gottumukkala Subba Raju.*)

omental patch. Caution should be exercised in using suction to close full-thickness perforations, especially in the colon because it risks entrapment of adjacent organs, including the bowel and ureter.

Over-the-Scope Clip Closure

Closure technique: over-the-scope clip device
The OTSC system, a super-elastic, nitinol, MRI conditional clip, is mounted on a clear distal cap at the end of an endoscope and is deployed using a mechanism similar to that used for band ligation. It results in a full-thickness closure by using teeth arranged in the shape of a bear trap.[16]

Principles of over-the-scope clip closure of perforation using a twin grasper

1. *Suction technique:* Align the lesion at a 6 to 12 o'clock position, if possible. Gentle and careful suction of the mucosal edges is appropriate to suction fresh edges of the perforation into the cap for successful deployment of the OTSC.[17] As noted, the suction technique creates a risk of adjacent structures.
2. *Retraction technique:* Grasp all layers of the gastrointestinal wall, including the serosa, with the Twin Grasper positioned in the center of each perforation edge. Withdraw the grasper with the tissue into the center of the distal cap to assure that the entire perforation site is retracted into the cap before the clip is released (**Fig. 6**). Caution: avoid capturing the Twin Grasper with the clip.

For larger defects or when OTSC deployment is misaligned, leaving partial defect, a second OTSC can be deployed adjacent to the first one to complete defect closure.[18,19]

Overstitch Endoscopic Suturing Closure

An overstitch suturing device can provide tissue approximation of large defects. The device is loaded on a double channel therapeutic endoscope and incorporates a curved suturing needle, which can be reloaded multiple times without scope withdrawal.

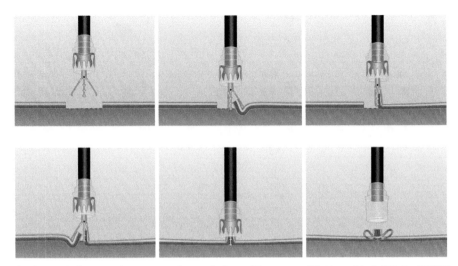

Fig. 6. OTSC closure using a retraction technique. (*Courtesy of* Gottumukkala S Raju, UT MD Anderson Cancer Center, Houston, Texas.)

Suturing is started at the furthest edge with placement of either continuous or interrupted sutures. One or 2 sets of sutures can be applied, depending on size and accessibility of defect. After the completion of each set of sutures, the anchor at the end of the suture is dropped and the suture is tightened to approximate the defect followed by cinching.[20]

Assessment of Transmural Injury and Prevention of Perforation

Endoscopic mucosal resection
Colonic perforation occurs in 1% to 2% of cases after EMR of laterally spreading tumors.[21,22] The incorporation of a blue dye (indigo carmine or methylene blue) into the submucosal injection solution has helped us to define the depth of resection. Submucosal connective tissue stains blue, whereas the muscularis propria and scar tissue do not take up the stain and appear white. Examination of resection base after every snare resection during EMR or widefield EMR is critical to identify perforation or precursor lesions of perforation.

- *Perforation or full-thickness transmural resection* needs immediate endoluminal closure or surgery.[23]
- *Partial or full-thickness muscularis propria resection*, identified by the target sign requires immediate clip closure because of risk of imminent perforation. Swan and colleagues[24] described the target sign, a marker of either partial or full-thickness muscularis propria resection, that is characterized by a white to gray circle of resected muscularis propria layer on the transected surface of the specimen surrounded by a web of blue-stained submucosal tissue and encircled by white cauterized mucosa. Clip closure of such defects avoids surgery.[22]
- *Unclear about the depth of resection*, submucosal chromoendoscopy helps to define the depth of resection; this process involves spraying indigo carmine-stained or methylene blue-stained saline solution on the resection base. Submucosa in the resection defect appears as a relatively homogenous blue mat of intersecting obliquely oriented submucosal connective tissue fiber. Muscle fibers and scar tissue do not take up the stain and appear as unstained areas.[25]

Whenever the depth of resection extends beyond the submucosa, clip closure of the defect is essential to avoid delayed perforation.

- *Sydney classification of deep mural injury:* Burgess and colleagues[22] recently proposed 5 types of deep mural injury after EMR, the Sydney classification, and suggested management based on the findings (**Fig. 7**). Deep mural injury is graded according to muscularis propria injury (I/II intact muscularis propria without or with fibrosis, III target sign, IV/V obvious transmural perforation without or with contamination). It is important to appreciate that the strongest layer in the colon wall is the submucosa. Whenever there is complete disruption of the submucosa and injury extends to the muscularis propria, it predisposes to delayed perforation; hence, use of this standardized system may aid in the selection of prophylactic clipping of those at risk for delayed perforations. **Fig. 8** shows a type 3 muscle injury occurring during EMR of a right colon lesion and its closure with hemostatic clips. The majority of the deep muscle injuries during EMR occur in the transverse colon and after en bloc resection of lesions and lesions with high-grade dysplasia or submucosal invasive cancer.[22]

Endoscopic submucosal dissection
The National Cancer Center in Japan reported a perforation rate of 2.4% in a series of 900 colorectal endoscopic submucosal dissections between 2004 and 2012.[26]

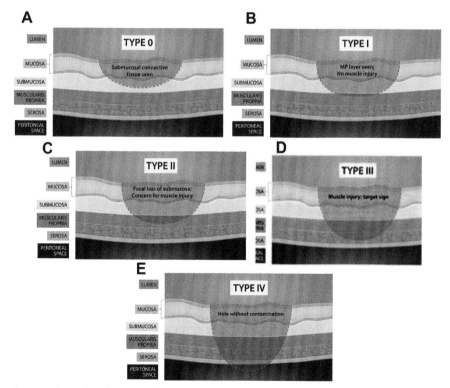

Fig. 7. Sydney classification of deep mural injury of the colon during EMR (A–E). MP, muscularis propria. (© *2019 Gottumukkala Subba Raju.*)

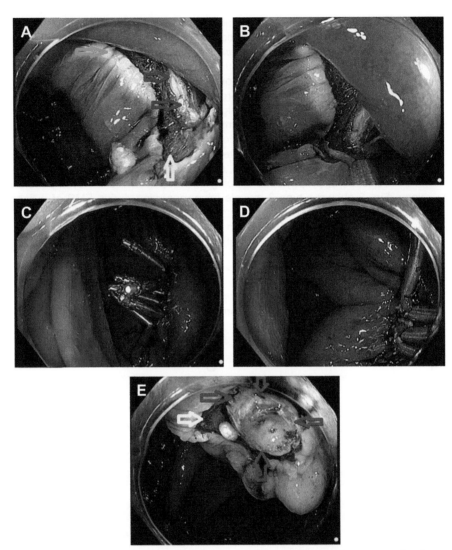

Fig. 8. Type 3 muscle injury and hemostatic clip closure after EMR of a 2-cm previously tat-tooed lesion on the ileocecal valve. (*A*) The submucosal defect (*yellow arrow*) is black because of previous tattoo placed under the lesion by the referring doctor. This tattoo might have contributed to the injury. The edge of the defect has a white cautery burn on it (*green arrow*). The thick white band (*red arrows*) is the cut edge of the muscle. The com-plete muscle injury is partly obscured by a fold of normal mucosa on the upper right. (*B*) The first clip is ready for placement at the lower edge of the muscle defect. (*C*) The fully closed defect. Note that the clips are placed close to each other. In this instance, the entire submu-cosal defect is closed but clips in general should be placed to fully close the muscle injury (*D*). After clip placement the colonoscope tip is moved to the proximal side of the clip line and the clips are deflected distally to check that the muscle injury is fully closed. (*E*) The underside of the specimen shows submucosa (*yellow arrow*) and a circle of white muscle (*red arrows*). (*Courtesy* Douglas K Rex, Indianapolis, IN.)

Outcome of Endoscopic Closure of Perforations

Benefits of endoscopic closure

- Successful endoscopic closure of perforations avoids surgery.
- TTSCs are successful in the closure of 90% of iatrogenic colon perforations.[27,28]
- OTSCs are successful in the closure of 90%–100% of iatrogenic colon perforations.[28–32]
- Endoscopic suturing is also successful in the closure of perforations complicating colonoscopic resection as shown in a report of 16 cases.[20]

Endoscopists performing colon EMR and endoscopic submucosal dissection must be trained to recognize the depth of transmural resection and be prepared to close the defect to prevent or treat perforation. One should keep the following factors in mind when choosing equipment for successful closure of perforations.

- TTSC are readily available, easy to deploy for both the endoscopist and the assisting technician, and are most effective for defects up to 25 mm in size.
- OTSC is preferred for larger perforations up to 3 cm and perforations with a fibrotic edge, which are not amenable to TTSC closure.

Limitations of Endoscopic Closure

- *TTSC*: Clip retention during follow-up colonoscopy after EMR can be seen in 4% to 8% of cases.[33] One should be aware of clip artifacts in the scars of approximately 1 in 3 large EMR sites closed by clips; these artifacts could be differentiated from polyps by the nodular elevations with normal mucosal pit pattern.[34,35]
- *OTSC*: Closure of defects on the right side of colon has lower success rates in comparison with the left side because of limitations in controlling the endoscope tip; in addition, left-sided diverticulosis may interfere with the insertion of endoscope loaded with an OTSC.[30] Vigorous suction could entrap adjacent viscera and small intestine in the clip.[36] To avoid this complication, select a cap that is adherent to the edges of the perforation and rehearse suction a few times to avoid entrapping the adjacent viscera. OTSC retention for a month or longer occurs in two-thirds of patients owing to its attachment to submucosa and muscularis propria. OTSC stays in situ and may interfere with follow-up examination of the resected site for local recurrence.[37] Recently, a novel device for fragmentation of the clip by applying an electrical direct current pulse at 2 opposing sides of the clip allows extraction of the OTSC.[38]

POSTOPERATIVE MANAGEMENT

It is not the perforation that kills people; it is the escape of fecal material into the peritoneal cavity that starts the cascade of sepsis and septic shock. Hence, it is important to manage complications related to feces and fluid escaping into peritoneal cavity, confirm successful closure with radiologic imaging, and be prepared for prompt surgical closure if perforation closure is not successful by consulting surgeons early.

A strategy for endoscopic management of perforation after endoluminal closure based on the best available scientific evidence is summarized here.[38,39]

- *Decompress a tension pneumoperitoneum*: Use a wide bore angiocath for decompression of abdomen, if there is abdominal distension and respiratory distress.
- *Antibiotics*: Broad spectrum intravenous antibiotics for aerobic and anerobic coverage.

> **Box 1**
> **Guidelines for the endoscopic unit quality officer on endoscopic management of colonoscopic perforations**
>
> Protocol for management of endoscopic perforation: Develop a written protocol in collaboration with radiologists and surgeons, similar to a stroke or heart attack management protocol
> > Step 1: Define procedures at high risk for perforation (EMR, endoscopic submucosal dissection, Balloon dilation, stent insertion).
> > Step 2: Implement management policy before the introduction of a high risk procedure in a practice.
> > Step 3: Endoscopy reports size and location of perforation; endoscopic closure used; air or carbon dioxide insufflation.
> > Step 4: Hospitalization and surgical consultation for no or failed endoscopic closure of perforation and in patients whose clinical condition is deteriorating.
>
> *Adapted from* Paspatis GA., Dumonceau J-M., Barthet M., et al. Diagnosis and management of iatrogenic endoscopic perforations: European Society of Gastrointestinal Endoscopy (ESGE) Position Statement. Endoscopy 2014;46(8):693–711.

- *Bowel rest*: Consider nasogastric tube decompression for patients with colonic perforations.
- *Blood work*: Complete blood count, international normalized ratio, basic metabolic profile, liver function tests, and an electrocardiogram.
- *Surgical consultation*: Preferably a colorectal surgeon for colorectal perforations.
- *Hospitalization*: Coordinate admission with medical and surgical team.
- *Imaging studies*: Computed tomography scan of the abdomen with rectal water-soluble contrast only. There is no need for intravenous contrast for perforation studies.

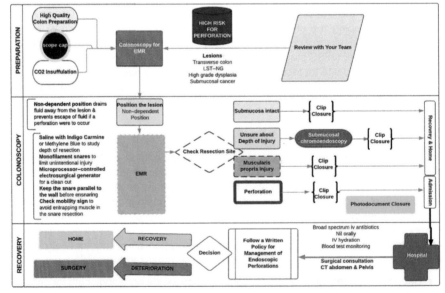

Fig. 9. Flow chart for prevention and management of colonoscopic resection defects and perforations. CT, computed tomography; IV, intravenous; LST-NG, laterally spreading tumor - non-granular type. (© 2019 Gottumukkala Subba Raju.)

- ○ *No leak*: Continue conservative management.
- ○ *Large leak*: Surgery.
- ○ *Small contained leak*: Options include continued conservative management, percutaneous drainage, or surgical repair, depending on the assessment of the multidisciplinary team.

Whether implementation of the strategy translates into improved clinical outcomes needs further investigation.

Institutional Protocol for Management of Endoscopic Perforations

The European Society for Gastrointestinal Endoscopy offers an excellent guidance on diagnosis and management of endoscopic perforations (**Box 1**; see **Fig. 1**).[23]

SUMMARY

Endoscopic closure of colonoscopic perforations is technically possible and prevents surgery. In addition, using safe EMR techniques will prevent deep resection and perforation. In addition, the identification of deep mural resection and prophylactic clip application prevents imminent perforations. Advances in endoluminal clip and suture closure have certainly helped endoscopists to resect large and complex polyps that once required surgery routinely (**Fig. 9**).

REFERENCES

1. Binmoeller KF, Grimm H, Soehendra N. Endoscopic closure of a perforation using metallic clips after snare excision of a gastric leiomyoma. Gastrointest Endosc 1993;39(2):172–4.
2. Yoshikane H, Hidano H, Sakakibara A, et al. Endoscopic repair by clipping of iatrogenic colonic perforation. Gastrointest Endosc 1997;46(5):464–6.
3. Mana F, De Vogelaere K, Urban D. Iatrogenic perforation of the colon during diagnostic colonoscopy: endoscopic treatment with clips. Gastrointest Endosc 2001; 54(2):258–9.
4. Raju GS, Pham B, Xiao S-Y, et al. A pilot study of endoscopic closure of colonic perforations with endoclips in a swine model. Gastrointest Endosc 2005;62(5):791–5.
5. Raju GS, Ahmed I, Xiao S-Y, et al. Controlled trial of immediate endoluminal closure of colon perforations in a porcine model by use of a novel clip device (with videos). Gastrointest Endosc 2006;64(6):989–97.
6. Raju GS, Ahmed I, Brining D, et al. Endoluminal closure of large perforations of colon with clips in a porcine model (with video). Gastrointest Endosc 2006;64(4):640–6.
7. Raju GS, Ahmed I, Shibukawa G, et al. Endoluminal clip closure of a circular full-thickness colon resection in a porcine model (with videos). Gastrointest Endosc 2007;65(3):503–9.
8. Raju GS, Fritscher-Ravens A, Rothstein RI, et al. Endoscopic closure of colon perforation compared to surgery in a porcine model: a randomized controlled trial (with videos). Gastrointest Endosc 2008;68(2):324–32.
9. Raju GS, Shibukawa G, Ahmed I, et al. Endoluminal suturing may overcome the limitations of clip closure of a gaping wide colon perforation (with videos). Gastrointest Endosc 2007;65(6):906–11.
10. Voermans RP, Vergouwe F, Breedveld P, et al. Comparison of endoscopic closure modalities for standardized colonic perforations in a porcine colon model. Endoscopy 2011;43:217–22.

11. von Renteln D, Kratt T, Rösch T, et al. Endoscopic full-thickness resection in the colon by using a clip-and-cut technique: an animal study. Gastrointest Endosc 2011;74(5):1108–14.

12. Raju GS, Malhotra A, Ahmed I. Colonoscopic full-thickness resection of the colon in a porcine model as a prelude to endoscopic surgery of difficult colon polyps: a novel technique (with videos). Gastrointest Endosc 2009;70(1):159–65.

13. Pham BV, Raju GS, Ahmed I, et al. Immediate endoscopic closure of colon perforation by using a prototype endoscopic suturing device: feasibility and outcome in a porcine model (with video). Gastrointest Endosc 2006;64(1):113–9.

14. Akimoto T, Goto O, Nishizawa T, et al. Endoscopic closure after intraluminal surgery. Dig Endosc 2017;29(5):547–58.

15. Ivekovic H, Vrzic D, Bilic B, et al. Release and re-hook: a novel method with combined use of clips and nylon snare to close a colonic defect after endoscopic mucosal resection. Endoscopy 2015;47:E545–6.

16. Matthes K, Jung Y, Kato M, et al. Efficacy of full-thickness GI perforation closure with a novel over-the-scope clip application device: an animal study. Gastrointest Endosc 2011;74(6):1369–75.

17. Donatelli G, Cereatti F, Dhumane P, et al. Closure of gastrointestinal defects with Ovesco clip: long-term results and clinical implications. Therap Adv Gastroenterol 2016;9(5):713–21.

18. Singhal S, Atluri S, Changela K, et al. Endoscopic closure of gastric perforation using over-the-scope clip: a surgery-sparing approach. Gastrointest Endosc 2014;79(1):23.

19. Kirtane T, Singhal S. Endoscopic closure of iatrogenic duodenal perforation using dual over-the-scope clips. Gastrointest Endosc 2016;83(2):467–8.

20. Kantsevoy SV, Bitner M, Hajiyeva G, et al. Endoscopic management of colonic perforations: clips versus suturing closure (with videos). Gastrointest Endosc 2016;84(3):487–93.

21. Moss A, Bourke MJ, Williams SJ, et al. Endoscopic mucosal resection outcomes and prediction of submucosal cancer from advanced colonic mucosal neoplasia. Gastroenterology 2011;140(7):1909–18.

22. Burgess NG, Bassan MS, McLeod D, et al. Deep mural injury and perforation after colonic endoscopic mucosal resection: a new classification and analysis of risk factors. Gut 2017;66(10):1779–89.

23. Paspatis GA, Dumonceau J-M, Barthet M, et al. Diagnosis and management of iatrogenic endoscopic perforations: European Society of Gastrointestinal Endoscopy (ESGE) position statement. Endoscopy 2014;46(8):693–711.

24. Swan MP, Bourke MJ, Moss A, et al. The target sign: an endoscopic marker for the resection of the muscularis propria and potential perforation during colonic endoscopic mucosal resection. Gastrointest Endosc 2011;73(1):79–85.

25. Holt BA, Jayasekeran V, Sonson R, et al. Topical submucosal chromoendoscopy defines the level of resection in colonic EMR and may improve procedural safety (with video). Gastrointest Endosc 2013;77(6):949–53.

26. Saito Y, Sakamoto T, Nakajima T, et al. Colorectal ESD: current indications and latest technical advances. Gastrointest Endosc Clin N Am 2014;24(2):245–55.

27. Mangiavillano B, Viaggi P, Masci E. Endoscopic closure of acute iatrogenic perforations during diagnostic and therapeutic endoscopy in the gastrointestinal tract using metallic clips: a literature review. J Dig Dis 2010;11(1):12–8.

28. Verlaan T, Voermans RP, van Berge Henegouwen MI, et al. Endoscopic closure of acute perforations of the GI tract: a systematic review of the literature. Gastrointest Endosc 2015;82(4):618–28.e5.

29. Voermans RP, Le Moine O, von Renteln D, et al. Efficacy of endoscopic closure of acute perforations of the gastrointestinal tract. Clin Gastroenterol Hepatol 2012; 10(6):603–8.
30. Gubler C, Bauerfeind P. Endoscopic closure of iatrogenic gastrointestinal tract perforations with the over-the-scope clip. Digestion 2012;85(4):302–7.
31. Hagel AF, Naegel A, Lindner AS, et al. Over-the-scope clip application yields a high rate of closure in gastrointestinal perforations and may reduce emergency surgery. J Gastrointest Surg 2012;16(11):2132–8.
32. Coriat R, Leblanc S, Pommaret E, et al. Endoscopic management of endoscopic submucosal dissection perforations: a new over-the-scope clip device. Gastrointest Endosc 2011;73(5):1067–9.
33. Ponugoti PL, Rex DK. Clip retention rates and rates of residual polyp at the base of retained clips on colorectal EMR sites. Gastrointest Endosc 2017;85(3):530–4.
34. Sreepati G, Vemulapalli KC, Rex DK. Clip artifact after closure of large colorectal EMR sites: incidence and recognition. Gastrointest Endosc 2015;82(2):344–9.
35. Pellisé M, Desomer L, Burgess NG, et al. The influence of clips on scars after EMR: clip artifact. Gastrointest Endosc 2016;83(3):608–16.
36. Loske G, Schorsch T, Daseking E, et al. Small intestine grasped by over-the-scope-clip during attempt to close an iatrogenic colonic perforation. Endoscopy 2016;48(S 01):E26–7.
37. Law R, Irani S, Wong Kee L, et al. Sa1481 clip retention following endoscopic placement of the over-the-scope clip (OTSC). Gastrointest Endosc 2013;77(5): AB221–2.
38. Caputo A, Schmidt A, Caca K, et al. Efficacy and safety of the remOVE System for OTSC® and FTRD® clip removal: data from a PMCF analysis. Minim Invasive Ther Allied Technol 2018;27(3):138–42.
39. Kowalczyk L, Forsmark CE, Ben-David K, et al. Algorithm for the management of endoscopic perforations: a quality improvement project. Am J Gastroenterol 2011;106(6):1022–7.

The Cold Revolution
How Far Can It Go?

Nicholas J. Tutticci, MBBS, FRACP[a,b,c],
Ammar O. Kheir, MBBS, MRCP, FRACP[a,b,c],
David G. Hewett, MBBS, MSc, PhD, FRACP[a,b,d],*

KEYWORDS

- Colorectal polyp • Polypectomy • Endoscopic mucosal resection • Cold snare
- Electrocautery • Colonoscopy

KEY POINTS

- Cold snare resection is remarkably safe, with comparably low complications for small polyps and for large polyps 10 to 60 mm.
- Cold snaring requires adoption of a piecemeal technique for polyps larger than 10 to 12 mm and a focus on inclusion of a margin of normal mucosa at the resection edge. For large polyps, the boundaries of resection are evolving; however, large sessile and pedunculated polyps are not suited to cold polypectomy.
- Cold snaring is efficacious for sessile serrated polyps regardless of size and the authors recommend a cold endoscopic mucosal resection (EMR) technique.
- The efficacy of cold polypectomy for adenomatous polyps is unknown. Studies using adjuvant cold forceps or thermal therapy report rates of residual neoplasia of 9% to 20%. Further research should clarify the efficacy of dedicated cold resection techniques and the suitability criteria of conventional adenomas for cold EMR.
- Cold snare resection is not recommended for endoscopic removal of known or suspected submucosal invasive adenocarcinoma because of its limited capacity to achieve submucosal resection depth.

Disclosure: D.G. Hewett has received research support from FujiFilm Australia and Olympus Corporation, and is a consultant for Boston Scientific and US Endoscopy. The other authors have nothing to disclose.

[a] Faculty of Medicine, The University of Queensland, Brisbane, Queensland, Australia; [b] Department of Gastroenterology, Queen Elizabeth II Jubilee Hospital, Cnr Kessels and Troughton Roads, Coopers Plains, Brisbane, Queensland 4108, Australia; [c] Digestive Disease Institute, Cleveland Clinic Abu Dhabi, Abu Dhabi, UAE; [d] Brisbane Colonoscopy, Brisbane, Queensland, Australia
* Corresponding author. Brisbane Colonoscopy, PO Box 267, Red Hill, Brisbane, Queensland 4059, Australia.
E-mail address: d.hewett@uq.edu.au
; @ammarkheir (A.O.K.); @dghewett (D.G.H.)

Gastrointest Endoscopy Clin N Am 29 (2019) 721–736
https://doi.org/10.1016/j.giec.2019.06.003
1052-5157/19/© 2019 Elsevier Inc. All rights reserved.

The last decade has seen the rapid emergence of cold resection techniques as the preferred modality for most colorectal polyps encountered at colonoscopy. The main advantage of cold resection techniques is enhanced safety, and this lack of risk has likely driven the rapid adoption into clinical practice. By omitting electrocautery, cold resection avoids the risk of thermal injury to the colon wall, which can lead to postpolypectomy syndrome, perforation, or delayed bleeding.[1] Cold snaring is also significantly quicker than hot snaring for many lesions,[2,3] avoiding the need to apply a grounding plate to the patient or connect the electrosurgical unit, both of which translate into cost savings.

The paradigm shift to cold resection has been facilitated by its inevitable natural appeal to both proceduralists and patients, and started well before the availability of clear data on its efficacy. More contentious, and possibly revolutionary, is the extension of cold resection techniques to large polyps. Albeit subject to significant measurement bias,[4] polyps are classified by size into diminutive (1–5 mm), small (6–10 mm), and large (>10 mm) categories.[5] For cold resection, the threshold of 10 mm is the size at which a fundamental shift in cold resection technique is required. Because of the limitations of mechanical transection without electrocautery, lesions larger than or equal to 10 mm require a piecemeal approach. This change in practice is significant and warrants careful evaluation with justifiable concern. Can cold resection be safely and effectively applied in a piecemeal fashion?

This article discusses:

- The fundamental differences between hot and cold snare resection
- The case for small and diminutive polyps
- Our approach for cold resection of polyps less than 10 mm
- Cold resection of large polyps and the evidence
- Candidate lesion criteria for cold resection of large lesions
- Our approach to piecemeal cold resection

THE PROS AND CONS OF ELECTROCAUTERY

Although technique and snare selection may differ from conventional polypectomy, the fundamental difference with cold snaring is the absence of electrocautery. Electrocautery adds 3 advantages to snare resection. First, electrocautery enables wider and deeper snare resections. It swiftly and readily achieves transection through nearly any volume of tissue with an associated deeper resection.[6] Second, it leaves a thermal penumbra around the defect in the colon wall, providing hypothetical insurance against any microscopic residual neoplasia.[7] Third, electrocautery typically secures immediate hemostasis.

However, these advantages conversely are the limitations of cold snare resection (**Table 1**). First, it is not possible to mechanically transect large volumes of tissue with a cold snare. The upper size limit is unknown and likely influenced by snare type and tissue characteristics, such as the proportion of entrapped mucosa versus submucosa. Practically, a 10-mm polyp with a 1-mm to 2-mm margin of normal mucosa becomes a 12-mm to 14-mm diameter of tissue resection, which the authors find the limit of reliable cold snare resection. The depth of resection is also less with smaller volumes of submucosa removed.[6] In studies of the cold snare defect, remnant muscularis mucosae is recognized, indicating incomplete mucosal layer resection.[8] This remnant implies that lesions with submucosal invasion are less likely to be completely resected by cold snare. The second limitation is the lack of thermal penumbra; a wider margin of normal mucosa must therefore be resected to ensure complete lesion removal. The third limitation is intraprocedural bleeding, which does not seem to be

Table 1
Advantages and disadvantages of cold resection for large polyps

Advantages	Disadvantages
• Less clinically significant postpolypectomy bleeding • Lower cost (probable but requires study for larger polyps) • Deep mural injury rare • Safety profile may allow cold EMR at the time of polyp detection rather than returning for a further dedicated EMR procedure • Avoidance of cost and time associated with prophylactic clip closure of EMR defect • Easier assessment of the EMR scar at surveillance without the presence of clip artifact	• Obligatory piecemeal resection of polyps of 10–20 mm may increase surveillance burden compared with en bloc conventional resection for similar-sized polyps • Advantage of ablative property in thermal penumbra in reducing residual is lost • Efficacy in early colorectal cancer questionable • Greater number of resected fragments for a given large lesion may impair histopathologic assessment

Abbreviation: EMR, endoscopic mucosal resection.

of major clinical importance because significant intraprocedural bleeding is uncommon in advanced cold resection.[9]

The advantages of electrocautery also convey significant risk. The larger tissue resection volume and depth increase the risk of deep thermal injury to the colonic wall and perforation. They also expose more submucosal blood vessels, which are partially coaptively closed by heat, leading to rates of clinically significant delayed postpolypectomy bleeding.[10–13] The unpredictable risk of delayed bleeding can be reduced with clip closure of the defect; however, this is incurs time and equipment costs.[14] In contrast, cold resection is associated with a negligible risk of perforation or of delayed bleeding, avoiding the need for costly prophylactic clip closure.

The potential cost benefits with cold resection are also relevant and require further evaluation. Cost savings occur through omission of a patient grounding electrode pad and time to connect the electrosurgical unit. The time savings described with diminutive cold snaring also come from avoiding submucosal injection,[3] although the authors advocate injection for piecemeal cold snaring.[15] However, piecemeal cold snaring does not require prophylactic clipping or adjuvant ablative thermal techniques (eg, snare tip soft coagulation).[16]

In addition, the quality of specimen for histologic analysis is a limitation of any piecemeal resection, which is compounded with cold snare resection. Piecemeal cold snare resection generates a higher number of resection fragments (of more shallow depth) for submission to pathology. This reduced quality might, hypothetically, reduce diagnostic accuracy for subtle, focal submucosal invasion, although the same concerns apply for piecemeal conventional endoscopic mucosal resection (EMR).[17]

THE CASE FOR DIMINUTIVE AND SMALL POLYPS

Cold snare polypectomy has become the standard of care for diminutive (1–5 mm) colorectal polyps, and is the recommended technique in current endoscopy guidelines.[1] Cold snaring is more effective and more efficient than cold forceps resection[18,19] and is virtually without risk. Like others,[20] it is our practice to avoid cold forceps and use cold snares for all diminutive lesions. The use of either hot snare or hot forceps for diminutive lesions should be abandoned because of unacceptably high risks of delayed bleeding, transmural injury, and incomplete resection.[21,22]

For small polyps (6–9 mm), the superior safety profile of cold snare resection is attractive; however, the evidence for its efficacy is less clear and guideline recommendations are not definitive.[1] Recent data now support the efficacy of cold snare polypectomy for lesions less than 10 mm.[2,23–25]

Because immediate bleeding can be visualized and treated, cold techniques can even be used safely in patients taking antiplatelet/anticoagulants. In studies in anticoagulated patients, cold snaring eliminated the risk of delayed bleeding compared with using electrocautery (14% to 0%).[26,27]

THE BASICS OF COLD SNARING

The technique of cold snare resection is fundamentally different from hot snare polypectomy, with the key steps of cold snaring shown in **Fig. 1**. The authors teach a staged approach as shown, and emphasize the need to align the lesion with the instrument channel, to anchor the tip of the snare catheter beyond the lesion, and to advance the snare catheter during snare closure. These maneuvers are of central importance to securing a margin of normal tissue around the resected lesion.

The efficacy of en bloc cold snaring is size dependent,[24,28] and likely limited by the cutting capacity of the snare for lesions of a certain upper size limit. Snare wire stiffness is also important to enable tissue capture via downward pressure during snare closure, preventing tissue slippage and snare wire bending to preserve the margin of normal tissue to achieve complete resection. Snare size is also relevant, with a small opening diameter required to enable sufficient force transmission from the handle.

So-called cold snare stall remains a practical challenge and occurs frequently with en bloc resection of large or bulky lesions. Our staged approach to cold snare stall is summarized in **Box 1** and is intended to allow degloving or release of entrapped submucosa without losing grip of the overlying mucosa to avoid incomplete resection.[21]

FROM SMALL TO LARGE: HOW FAR CAN THIS TECHNIQUE GO?

The safety of cold snare resection is so alluring that expansion of cold snare resection to larger lesions is, in our view, inevitable. It is in these larger lesions, in which the risks of conventional EMR with electrocautery are magnified, that the greatest advantage of cold resection could be realized.

How large can this technique go? As highlighted by cold snare stall, the key size limitation of cold snaring is the capacity to efficiently transect larger fragments of tissue without failing to cut. Without electrocautery, en bloc transection of polyps approaching 10 mm with a mandatory margin of normal mucosa is difficult, if not impossible, for even larger polyps. At some threshold, piecemeal resection is required to avoid the need for electrocautery. The conventional approach for piecemeal resection has been the application of electrocautery for thermal eradication of neoplastic tissue at the margins of snare resection, which also allows a larger fragment size, with the upper size threshold for en bloc conventional EMR of 20 mm.[29] Piecemeal EMR with electrocautery permits removal of very large and even circumferential colonic neoplasia.[30,31]

With further evolution of cold resection techniques, electrocautery may not be required. Cold EMR is a simple modification of the conventional EMR technique,

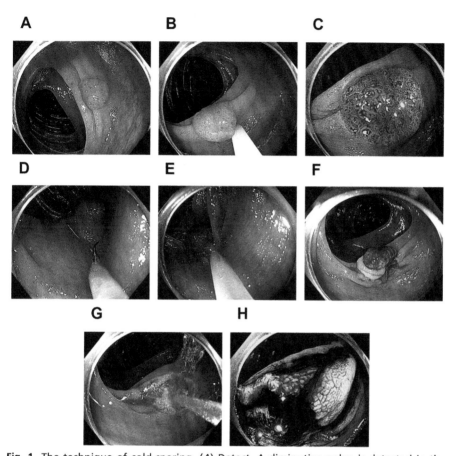

Fig. 1. The technique of cold snaring. (*A*) Detect. A diminutive polyp is detected in the transverse colon at the 2 o'clock position. (*B*) Align and measure. The insertion tube is rotated to align the polyp with the instrument channel (5–6 o'clock); the lesion size (7–8 mm) is measured by comparison with the snare catheter tip (2.6 mm). (*C*) Optical diagnosis. Image enhancement with narrow-band imaging (NBI) and optical magnification: Narrow-band Imaging International Colorectal Endoscopic (NICE) 2 with high confidence, indicating an adenoma. (*D*) Open and anchor. The snare is opened and positioned to capture the lesion and a margin of normal tissue. The catheter is then anchored distal to the lesion, by advancing the catheter while angling the instrument tip down and right. (*E*) Close and cut. Snare closure and transection while advancing the catheter and maintaining downward pressure. (*F*) Retrieve. After transection, the lesion remains within the defect for easy suction; note generous margin of normal tissue on left. (*G*) Wash. Washing of defect to expand submucosal space. (*H*) Inspect. The margin of the defect is inspected with NBI and optical magnification (particularly on right side of defect where the margin was less generous) to ensure complete resection and absence of bleeding (minor bleeding is typical).

requiring conventional snare resection to be applied consistently and repeatedly over the entire lesion, but without electrocautery. The lesion, with a wide margin, is simply removed in multiple, smaller pieces. So why should there be a size limit to piecemeal cold snare resection when no such arbitrary barrier is now applied to conventional EMR?

Box 1
Proposed cold snare stall technique

- Larger volumes of submucosal tissue capture can result in cold snare stall; this should be carefully managed to avoid incomplete resection.

- If the snare fails to transect with full closure, do not apply electrocautery; simply pause and begin stage 1 maneuvers. The authors strongly advise against electrocautery at this point.

- Stage 1: maximize force transmission down the snare wire:
  ○ Maintain insufflation and snare closure, and wait; slow transection may occur.
  ○ Reduce any loops in the instrument, and reduce angulation in the instrument tip.
  ○ Straighten the length of snare catheter from outside the scope to the snare handle.
  ○ Move the catheter back and forth within the instrument channel.

- After a few seconds, transection may occur. If not:

- Stage 2: release entrapped submucosa[a]:
  ○ Partially reopen the snare (up to one-third of the snare handle).
  ○ Gently lift or tent the lesion away from the wall and watch for release of the stalk of submucosa (analogous to repositioning the snare further up the stalk of a pedunculated polyp).
  ○ Lower the lesion.
  ○ Close the snare fully again.

- The tip of the cold snare polypectomy defect stalk or protrusion always requires endoscopic interrogation. If there is any concern about residual neoplasia at the tip, the authors recommend repeat cold snare resection of the distal end of the protrusion.

[a] The partially transected tissue generally has the configuration of a mushroom in which the cap is the mucosal layer containing the polyp and the stem is bunched up submucosa trapped within the closed snare wire. Transection requires mucosal release or degloving around the entrapped submucosa.

WHAT IS THE EVIDENCE FOR COLD ENDOSCOPIC MUCOSAL RESECTION?

The consistent finding of all studies of cold resection for larger polyps, regardless of the use of submucosal injection, is safety (**Table 2**). Intraprocedural bleeding is uncommon and easily treated. Postprocedure adverse events are rare and overall comparable with those described for cold snaring of small polyps.[2] However, safety alone is not enough, but existing data on the efficacy of cold resection are limited, observational, and heterogeneous, likely reflecting lesion selection and cold resection technique.

Two prospective observational studies have evaluated cold snare resection of large sessile serrated polyps (SSPs).[15,32] The authors recently published a large series of piecemeal cold EMR (10–40 mm),[15] whereas Tate and colleagues[32] reported a series of piecemeal resection without injection (10–35 mm). Both are from high-volume academic endoscopy centers and show impressive efficacy outcomes. In our study, margin biopsies were positive in only 2 lesions (1.2%) and, on surveillance within 12 months, only 1 lesion had residual serrated neoplasia. Contrast this with the Complete Adenoma Resection (CARE) study of conventional hot snare polypectomy (up to 20 mm), in which incomplete resection was documented in nearly 50% of serrated lesions greater than 10 mm based on defect biopsies.[33] Further retrospective data from the United Kingdom also focused on SSPs alone, and showed a high complete resection rate.[34]

The case for cold resection of large serrated lesions is strong; however, data to support efficacy for conventional adenomas are very limited. Only 2 studies have reported

Table 2
Summary of observational studies of cold snare polypectomy for large (≥10 mm) polyps

Study	Technique	N	Size Range (mm)	Histology	Intraprocedural Bleeding Requiring Intervention	Adverse Events	Complete Surveillance (%)	Residual Neoplasia (%)
Tutticci & Hewett,[15] 2018 Prospective Australia	Cold EMR	163	10–40	SSP	1	3: Pain (1) minor bleeding not requiring medication attention (2)	82	0.6
Tate et al,[32] 2018 Prospective Australia	Piecemeal cold snare without injection	41	10–35	SSP	0	0	37	0
Rameshshanker et al,[34] 2018 Retrospective UK	Cold EMR	29	10–30	SSP	0	0	100	3.4
Piraka et al,[35] 2017 Retrospective United States	Cold EMR + adjuvant cold forceps in 29%	94	12–60	Unselected	1	0	77	9.7 (all adenomatous)
Muniraj et al,[36] 2015 Retrospective United States	Cold EMR + APC in 30%	30	10–30	Unselected	NA APC applied for ooze	0	90	20
Augusto Barros et al,[47] 2014 Retrospective Argentina	Piecemeal cold snare without injection	43	10–20	Unselected	0	1 (pain)	NA	NA

Abbreviations: APC, argon plasma coagulation; NA, not available; SSP, sessile serrated polyp.

on surveillance outcomes in cohorts of both serrated and conventional adenomatous lesions and residual neoplasia rates of 9.7% and 20% were seen, with the 9.7% recurrence rate entirely adenomatous.[35,36] However, in both these studies, adjunctive therapy (beyond cold snare) was applied in 30% of lesions (see **Table 2**: either biopsy forceps or argon plasma coagulation [APC]), suggesting that the primary snare resection was inadequate. Cold forceps resection applied piecemeal is less effective than cold snare, and adjuvant APC in conventional EMR is associated with higher rates of residual neoplasia, and it is possible that application of a pure snare resection technique may be more efficacious.[18,37,38]

The higher rates of residual adenoma seen after cold EMR compared with SSPs may therefore not be caused by biology but by the polypectomy technique. The presence of residual adenoma is likely caused by failure of the endoscopist to recognize lesion extent, resulting in marginal residual adenoma or, more likely, failure to ensure an adequate margin of normal mucosa during snare closure leading to marginal microresidual or island microresidual adenoma within the defect. The contribution of cold snare stall is also possible, and needs further evaluation. Techniques for responding to snare stall vary,[28] and the potential for submucosal remnant protrusion as a source of residual mucosal tissue in resection of large polyps, in contrast with small polyps, must be considered.[8]

Furthermore, even if cold EMR for adenomas is less effective than for SSPs, this does not mean failure, particularly when safety is a primary objective. It is well established that rates of residual neoplasia after conventional EMR are 15% to 20%, and higher than for SSPs matched for size.[39] Conventional EMR produces a lower rate of residual neoplasia for SSPs compared with adenomas (7% vs 28% respectively). Adenomatous histology is known to be an independent predictor of histologic recurrence (hazard ratio, 1.7).[40]

The presence of residual adenoma at correctly timed surveillance is a primary research end point but may have little clinical impact on long-term cure. In none of the cold resection studies (see **Table 2**) was any treatment beyond endoscopic therapy (eg, surgery) required to treat residual disease. However, only 1 study reported on completed clear surveillance after treatment of residual adenoma. Endoscopic residual neoplasia after conventional EMR is usually unifocal, diminutive, and readily treated endoscopically in more than 93% of cases, prompting calls for a shift to judge efficacy not at but after first surveillance and any residual polyp therapy.[39]

WHICH LARGE LESIONS ARE MOST SUITED TO COLD ENDOSCOPIC MUCOSAL RESECTION?

Like conventional approaches to colorectal resection, lesion selection is critical to the choice of resection technique.

SSPs are ideal candidate lesions for piecemeal cold snare resection. These lesions are flat and soft, and easily transected in multiple small pieces with a dedicated cold snare (9–10 mm). They are often numerous and located in the proximal colon, factors that are known to increase the risk for complications from conventional EMR. Safety and efficacy data for cold resection of SSPs are strong, at least when performed in expert centers. The authors recommend cold EMR for large SSPs if the endoscopist's skill and experience permit.[15]

Selected conventional adenomas are also likely suitable for cold EMR. For example, ideal lesions are those at low risk of submucosal invasion; for example, granular homogeneous Paris 0-IIa laterally spreading lesions with a Narrow-band Imaging International Colorectal Endoscopic (NICE) type 2 mucosal pattern.[37,41] In our experience, lateral lesion size is not a factor in lesion selection for cold EMR, because the fundamental technique of piecemeal resection is independent of lesion lateral extent. Extensive, even circumferential, lesions can be cured by conventional piecemeal EMR and the same principles apply to cold EMR.[30]

Some lesions are not suitable for cold resection. Candidate exclusion criteria for cold EMR include:

- Suspected submucosal invasion, for which en bloc endoscopic resection or surgical resection should be performed
- Large pedunculated polyps, for which tissue transection through a thick stalk will be unlikely and/or lead to significant immediate bleeding
- Large, sessile polyps with substantial tissue bulk, which may not transect with a cold snare and for which there is a higher risk of submucosal invasion

Lesion location may also be a consideration, such as the anal verge, where bleeding occurs more frequently, and although cold resection is feasible, persistent ooze would require either a clip in a location unpleasant for the patient or the use of electrocautery, diminishing the advantages of cold resection.

The main disadvantage of any form of piecemeal resection (hot or cold) is the limitation with histologic evaluation of a piecemeal specimen.[17,42] Piecemeal resection when invasive cancer is suspected may not allow accurate assessment for histopathologic staging and is not recommended. Therefore, nonpedunculated sessile or flat lesions should be carefully assessed endoscopically for signs of deep submucosally invasive cancer (before commencing resection). These features include lesion morphology (nongranular, depressed lesions) and mucosal patterns. Deep submucosal cancers can be identified reliably as type 3 lesions using the NICE classification with characteristic disruption and loss of mucosal vascular and surface patterns.[17,43,44] Lesions with deep submucosal invasive cancer should not be resected endoscopically. Arguably, lesions with suspected superficial invasion should be removed en bloc, and not with piecemeal resection; however, current image-enhancement technologies, even with magnification, cannot reliably distinguish superficial submucosal invasion from high-grade dysplasia.

Box 2
Unanswered research questions for cold snare resection

- Is submucosal injection required for cold snare resection of large polyps?
- What are the ideal constituents of the submucosal injectate for cold snaring (crystalloid vs colloid, need for chromic dye or epinephrine)?
- What are the ideal snare characteristics for piecemeal cold snare resection? Are further refinements in snare design possible to improve tissue capture and cutting performance?
- What lesions are suitable for piecemeal cold snare resection?
- Can piecemeal cold snare resection be safely and effectively applied without cessation of antiplatelet/anticoagulants?
- What are the endoscopic characteristics of the cold EMR scar for localization and diagnosis of residual neoplasia?
- Can cold snare resection be used to treat residual neoplasia after index cold EMR (see **Fig. 5**)?
- What is the best measure of polypectomy effectiveness?
- What is the best method for measuring the complete resection rate? How should completeness of resection be assessed in real time, immediately after polypectomy?
- What technique should be applied for cold snare stall (when the snare fails to cold resect)?

In addition, some patients are more suited to cold resection techniques independent of the target polyp. For example, the authors prefer cold resection for patients in whom the risks of electrocautery are magnified, such as those remaining on or resuming anti-coagulant/antiplatelet agents, those patient with comorbidities that would least tolerate electrocautery complications, or those patients returning to remote locations for whom access to specialist endoscopy is limited. In our view, the advantages of cold EMR are more significant in these contexts and should factor in selection of resection technique. Ultimately, we envisage a combined patient-based and lesion-based approach to endo-scopic resection for large lesions using the full spectrum from cold EMR through con-ventional EMR to endoscopic submucosal dissection.

OPTIMAL COLD ENDOSCOPIC MUCOSAL RESECTION TECHNIQUE: OUR APPROACH

Optimal techniques of cold resection remain unclear. Unresolved questions (**Box 2**) concern the role, requirement for, and type of submucosal injection, and the use of adjuvant resection or ablative techniques (biopsy forceps or thermal therapies). Our approach and preferred technique of cold EMR without adjuvant therapy are described here (**Box 3, Figs. 2–5**).

Based on technical rationale and our study of efficacy in large SSPs, we recom-mend the routine use of submucosal injection before cold resection of large polyps.[15] We find submucosal injection containing a contrast dye very helpful for delineating lesion margins, particularly for SSPs. Contrast injection, together with

---

Box 3
Tips for optimal cold endoscopic mucosal resection technique

- Include dilute indigo carmine or methylene blue in the injectate to help define the lesion.
- The addition of epinephrine is not recommended.
- Inject and elevate the entire lesion before resection.
- Commence at margin and aim for 30% to 50% of tissue resection to be endoscopically normal mucosa.
- Limit the diameter of each tissue fragment to less than 10 mm for each resection.
- Suction each resected fragment after transection (without removing the snare from the instrument channel; the fragments are small enough to suction around the catheter).
- For adenomatous lesions larger than 30 mm consider submitting specimens in 2 or more pathology jars.
- Interrogate the resection margin and defect and perform repeated cold EMR for any areas of suspicion for residual neoplasia. Polyp islands within the defect can be safely removed by targeted resection with a partially opened snare.
- Do not apply thermal therapy empirically to the defect margin; the efficacy and safety of this approach have been studied in conventional EMR but not cold EMR.
- When snare stall occurs, do not apply electrocautery but relax the snare partially, reposition further up the stalk/protrusion and away from the wall without loss of captured mucosa before resnaring (see **Box 1**).
- If there is persistent bleeding (which is unusual), targeted application of a clip is preferred to thermal therapy. If hemostasis is achieved with a single clip, then clip closure of the entire lesion is not necessary.

From Tutticci NJ, Hewett DG. Cold EMR of large sessile serrated polyps at colonoscopy (with video). Gastrointest Endosc 2018;87:837-842; with permission.

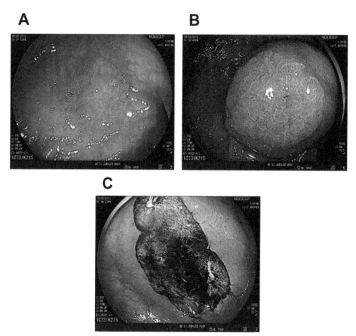

Fig. 2. Cold EMR of a large sessile serrated polyp. (*A*) A 15-mm ascending colon SSP with indistinct borders. (*B*) Improved delineation of the entire lesion after submucosal injection with indigo carmine and succinylated gelatin without epinephrine. (*C*) Final cold EMR defect.

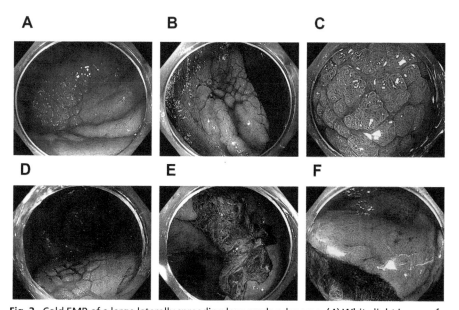

Fig. 3. Cold EMR of a large laterally spreading low-grade adenoma. (*A*) White light image of a 40-mm granular laterally spreading adenoma in the proximal ascending colon. (*B*) After application of topical indigo carmine: Paris 0-IIa. (*C*) Detailed interrogation of the entire lesion under NBI with optical magnification: NICE 2 throughout. (*D*) Submucosal injection to elevate the entire lesion (indigo carmine with succinylated gelatin without epinephrine). (*E*) Final cold EMR defect. (*F*) Interrogation of defect margin under NBI with optical magnification.

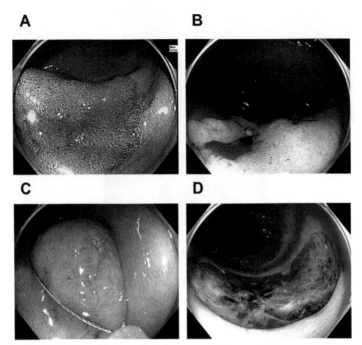

Fig. 4. Cold EMR of a large high-grade adenoma. A 25-mm mid–transverse colon nongranular adenoma with high-grade dysplasia was referred for endoscopic resection following biopsy. (*A*) Detailed interrogation of the entire lesion under NBI with optical magnification: NICE 2 throughout. (*B*) Submucosal injection produced only partial central elevation because of biopsy-related submucosal fibrosis. (*C*) Cold EMR commencing at lesion margin including clear margin of normal mucosa. (*D*) Final cold EMR defect showing central fibrosis.

high-definition imaging, is invaluable for recognition of residual neoplasia, particularly with remnant serrated pits in SSPs. Injection also facilitates access to larger lesions (such as those proximal to or within haustral folds) and for improving the ease of tissue transection. In our anecdotal experience, we find that injection reduces the rates of cold snare stall and the associated remnant cords or protrusions after transection.

Studies to define the optimal injectate are needed. Colloidal injectate is advocated for conventional EMR because a sustained submucosal lift facilitates a quicker resection in fewer pieces.[45] However, cold EMR is so rapid that a saline-based injectate may be just as effective. We find inclusion of a contrast agent, such as indigo carmine or methylene blue, important; however, the optimal concentration is unknown. The addition of dilute epinephrine maintains a bloodless resection field; however, in our experience it is of limited benefit because immediate bleeding is mostly minimal and short lived.[15] In conventional EMR, dilute epinephrine is routinely included, although its benefit, if any, seems to be in reducing delayed bleeding.[11,12]

In addition, studies have attempted to define the optimal snare for cold EMR where wire traction to achieve tissue capture and a thin wire for easy transection are both desirable attributes (see **Table 2**). The emergence of dedicated cold snares is welcome, given their proven benefit compared with conventional snares for use with electrocautery.[28,46] However, the snare performance required for cold EMR

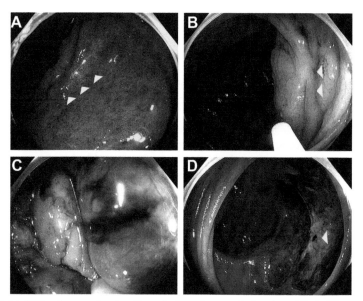

Fig. 5. Cold EMR of a previously attempted sessile serrated polyp. (*A*) A 35-mm residual ascending colon sessile serrated polyp after previous attempt with central scar (*yellow arrows*). (*B*) Limited lifting of central scar area (*arrows*). (*C*) Cold EMR of entire lesion with tissue capture of central scarred area for cold EMR aided by cap suction technique and thin wire snare. (*D*) Cold EMR defect with central scar and tethering apparent. No adverse events recorded and no residual neoplasia identified at first surveillance.

may be different from that required for small and diminutive polyps. The target lesion with cold EMR can be tense, tented, and difficult to capture/ensnare, a very different snare environment to cold resection without injectate. Therefore, mucosal traction may be more important for large lesions, and, for patients with multiple large lesions, snare durability can become a factor.

SUMMARY: THE COLD REVOLUTION

As an emerging technique for large and noninvasive colorectal neoplasia, piecemeal cold resection is overwhelmingly safe and promises to eliminate the hazards of conventional resection with electrocautery. Preliminary data on efficacy are extremely promising, particularly for SSPs in expert centers. The efficacy of cold piecemeal resection for conventional adenomas requires further observational study and randomized trials to compare residual rates and cost savings, and enable a lesion-specific approach. Further questions remain about the optimal technique, including use and choice of injectate, snare design, and selection.

The potential widespread adoption of cold EMR in the colorectum is a revolution. Although the authors advocate caution with lesion selection when invasive cancer is suspected, the potential cost savings of cold resection, compared with conventional EMR, through avoidance of clip closure and delayed bleeding, and cessation of antiplatelets/anticoagulants, will have substantial impact. For selected lesions, there may be no upper size limit, and the technique promises major gains in safety, efficiency, and cost-effectiveness of cancer prevention at colonoscopy.

REFERENCES

1. Ferlitsch M, Moss A, Hassan C, et al. Colorectal polypectomy and endoscopic mucosal resection (EMR): European Society of Gastrointestinal Endoscopy (ESGE) clinical guideline. Endoscopy 2017;49:270–97.
2. Ichise Y, Horiuchi A, Nakayama Y, et al. Prospective randomized comparison of cold snare polypectomy and conventional polypectomy for small colorectal polyps. Digestion 2011;84:78–81.
3. Paspatis GA, Tribonias G, Konstantinidis K, et al. A prospective randomized comparison of cold vs hot snare polypectomy in the occurrence of postpolypectomy bleeding in small colonic polyps. Colorectal Dis 2011;13:e345–8.
4. Sakata S, McIvor F, Klein K, et al. Measurement of polyp size at colonoscopy: a proof-of-concept simulation study to address technology bias. Gut 2018;67:206–8.
5. Chaptini L, Chaaya A, Depalma F, et al. Variation in polyp size estimation among endoscopists and impact on surveillance intervals. Gastrointest Endosc 2014;80:652–9.
6. Suzuki S, Gotoda T, Kusano C, et al. Width and depth of resection for small colorectal polyps: hot versus cold snare polypectomy. Gastrointest Endosc 2018;87:1095–103.
7. Takayanagi D, Nemoto D, Isohata N, et al. Histological comparison of cold versus hot snare resections of the colorectal mucosa. Dis Colon Rectum 2018;61:964–70.
8. Tutticci N, Burgess NG, Pellise M, et al. Characterization and significance of protrusions in the mucosal defect after cold snare polypectomy. Gastrointest Endosc 2015;82(3):523–8.
9. Thoguluva Chandrasekar V, Spadaccini M, Aziz M, et al. Cold snare endoscopic resection of nonpedunculated colorectal polyps larger than 10 mm: a systematic review and pooled-analysis. Gastrointest Endosc 2019;89(5):929–36.e3.
10. Yamashina T, Fukuhara M, Maruo T, et al. Cold snare polypectomy reduced delayed postpolypectomy bleeding compared with conventional hot polypectomy: a propensity score-matching analysis. Endosc Int Open 2017;5:E587–94.
11. Bahin FF, Rasouli KN, Byth K, et al. Prediction of clinically significant bleeding following wide-field endoscopic resection of large sessile and laterally spreading colorectal lesions: a clinical risk score. Am J Gastroenterol 2016;111:1115–22.
12. Burgess NG, Metz AJ, Williams SJ, et al. Risk factors for intraprocedural and clinically significant delayed bleeding after wide-field endoscopic mucosal resection of large colonic lesions. Clin Gastroenterol Hepatol 2014;12:651–61.e1-3.
13. Metz AJ, Bourke MJ, Moss A, et al. Factors that predict bleeding following endoscopic mucosal resection of large colonic lesions. Endoscopy 2011;43:506–11.
14. Pohl H, Grimm IS, Moyer MT, et al. Clip closure prevents bleeding after endoscopic resection of large colon polyps in a randomized trial. Gastroenterology 2019. https://doi.org/10.1053/j.gastro.2019.03.019.
15. Tutticci NJ, Hewett DG. Cold EMR of large sessile serrated polyps at colonoscopy (with video). Gastrointest Endosc 2018;87:837–42.
16. Klein A, Tate DJ, Jayasekeran V, et al. Thermal ablation of mucosal defect margins reduces adenoma recurrence after colonic endoscopic mucosal resection. Gastroenterology 2019;156:604–13.e3.
17. Hewett DG, Sakata S. Classifications for optical diagnosis of colorectal lesions: not 2B with JNET. Gastrointest Endosc 2017;85:822–8.

18. Kim JS, Lee BI, Choi H, et al. Cold snare polypectomy versus cold forceps polypectomy for diminutive and small colorectal polyps: a randomized controlled trial. Gastrointest Endosc 2015;81:741–7.

19. Park SK, Ko BM, Han JP, et al. A prospective randomized comparative study of cold forceps polypectomy by using narrow-band imaging endoscopy versus cold snare polypectomy in patients with diminutive colorectal polyps. Gastrointest Endosc 2016;83:527–32.

20. Rex DK, Dekker E. How we resect colorectal polyps <20 mm in size. Gastrointest Endosc 2019;89:449–52.

21. Hewett DG. Cold snare polypectomy: optimizing technique and technology (with videos). Gastrointest Endosc 2015;82:693–6.

22. Hewett DG. Colonoscopic polypectomy: current techniques and controversies. Gastroenterol Clin North Am 2013;42:443–58.

23. Kawamura T, Takeuchi Y, Asai S, et al. A comparison of the resection rate for cold and hot snare polypectomy for 4-9 mm colorectal polyps: a multicentre randomised controlled trial (CRESCENT study). Gut 2018;67:1950–7.

24. Papastergiou V, Paraskeva KD, Fragaki M, et al. Cold versus hot endoscopic mucosal resection for nonpedunculated colorectal polyps sized 6-10 mm: a randomized trial. Endoscopy 2018;50:403–11.

25. Zhang Q, Gao P, Han B, et al. Polypectomy for complete endoscopic resection of small colorectal polyps. Gastrointest Endosc 2018;87:733–40.

26. Horiuchi A, Nakayama Y, Kajiyama M, et al. Removal of small colorectal polyps in anticoagulated patients: a prospective randomized comparison of cold snare and conventional polypectomy. Gastrointest Endosc 2014;79:417–23.

27. Arimoto J, Chiba H, Ashikari K, et al. Safety of cold snare polypectomy in patients receiving treatment with antithrombotic agents. Dig Dis Sci 2019. https://doi.org/10.1007/s10620-019-5469-1.

28. Horiuchi A, Hosoi K, Kajiyama M, et al. Prospective, randomized comparison of 2 methods of cold snare polypectomy for small colorectal polyps. Gastrointest Endosc 2015;82:686–92.

29. Nanda KS, Bourke MJ. Endoscopic mucosal resection and complications. Tech Gastrointest Endosc 2013;15:88–95.

30. Tutticci N, Klein A, Sonson R, et al. Endoscopic resection of subtotal or completely circumferential laterally spreading colonic adenomas: technique, caveats, and outcomes. Endoscopy 2016;48:465–71.

31. Tutticci N, Sonson R, Bourke MJ. Endoscopic resection of subtotal and complete circumferential colonic advanced mucosal neoplasia. Gastrointest Endosc 2014;80:340.

32. Tate DJ, Awadie H, Bahin FF, et al. Wide-field piecemeal cold snare polypectomy of large sessile serrated polyps without a submucosal injection is safe. Endoscopy 2018;50:248–52.

33. Pohl H, Srivastava A, Bensen SP, et al. Incomplete polyp resection during colonoscopy: results of the Complete Adenoma Resection (CARE) study. Gastroenterology 2013;144:74–80 e1.

34. Rameshshanker R, Tsiamoulos Z, Latchford A, et al. Resection of large sessile serrated polyps by cold piecemeal endoscopic mucosal resection: serrated COld Piecemeal Endoscopic mucosal resection (SCOPE). Endoscopy 2018;50:E165–7.

35. Piraka C, Saeed A, Waljee AK, et al. Cold snare polypectomy for nonpedunculated colon polyps greater than 1 cm. Endosc Int Open 2017;5:E184–9.

36. Muniraj T, Sahakian A, Ciarleglio MM, et al. Cold snare polypectomy for large sessile colonic polyps: a single-center experience. Gastroenterol Res Pract 2015;2015:175959.

37. Moss A, Bourke MJ, Williams SJ, et al. Endoscopic mucosal resection outcomes and prediction of submucosal cancer from advanced colonic mucosal neoplasia. Gastroenterology 2011;140:1909–18.

38. Lee CK, Shim JJ, Jang JY. Cold snare polypectomy vs. Cold forceps polypectomy using double-biopsy technique for removal of diminutive colorectal polyps: a prospective randomized study. Am J Gastroenterol 2013;108:1593–600.

39. Moss A, Williams SJ, Hourigan LF, et al. Long-term adenoma recurrence following wide-field endoscopic mucosal resection (WF-EMR) for advanced colonic mucosal neoplasia is infrequent: results and risk factors in 1000 cases from the Australian Colonic EMR (ACE) study. Gut 2015;64:57–65.

40. Pellise M, Burgess NG, Tutticci N, et al. Endoscopic mucosal resection for large serrated lesions in comparison with adenomas: a prospective multicentre study of 2000 lesions. Gut 2017;66:644–53.

41. Burgess NG, Hourigan LF, Zanati SA, et al. Risk stratification for covert invasive cancer among patients referred for colonic endoscopic mucosal resection: a large multicenter cohort. Gastroenterology 2017;153:732–42.

42. Sakata S, Kheir AO, Hewett DG. Optical diagnosis of colorectal neoplasia: a western perspective. Dig Endosc 2016;28:281–8.

43. Hayashi N, Tanaka S, Hewett DG, et al. Endoscopic prediction of deep submucosal invasive carcinoma: validation of the narrow-band imaging international colorectal endoscopic (NICE) classification. Gastrointest Endosc 2013;78:625–32.

44. Puig I, Lopez-Ceron M, Arnau A, et al. Accuracy of the narrow-band imaging international colorectal endoscopic classification system in identification of deep invasion in colorectal polyps. Gastroenterology 2019;156:75–87.

45. Moss A, Bourke MJ, Metz AJ. A randomized, double-blind trial of succinylated gelatin submucosal injection for endoscopic resection of large sessile polyps of the colon. Am J Gastroenterol 2010;105:2375–82.

46. Dwyer JP, Tan JYC, Urquhart P, et al. A prospective comparison of cold snare polypectomy using traditional or dedicated cold snares for the resection of small sessile colorectal polyps. Endosc Int Open 2017;5:E1062–8.

47. Augusto Barros R, Monteverde M, Federico Barros R, et al. [Safety and efficacy of cold snare resection of non-polypoid colorectal lesions (0-IIa and 0-IIb)]. Acta Gastroenterol Latinoam 2014;44:27–32.

UNITED STATES POSTAL SERVICE ® Statement of Ownership, Management, and Circulation
(All Periodicals Publications Except Requester Publications)

1. Publication Title	2. Publication Number	3. Filing Date
GASTROINTESTINAL ENDOSCOPY CLINICS OF NORTH AMERICA	012 – 603	9/18/2019

4. Issue Frequency	5. Number of Issues Published Annually	6. Annual Subscription Price
JAN, APR, JUL, OCT	4	$359.00

7. Complete Mailing Address of Known Office of Publication *(Not printer) (Street, city, county, state, and ZIP+4®)*

ELSEVIER INC.
230 Park Avenue, Suite 800
New York, NY 10169

Contact Person
STEPHEN R. BUSHING

Telephone *(Include area code)*
215-239-3688

8. Complete Mailing Address of Headquarters or General Business Office of Publisher *(Not printer)*

ELSEVIER INC.
230 Park Avenue, Suite 800
New York, NY 10169

9. Full Names and Complete Mailing Addresses of Publisher, Editor, and Managing Editor *(Do not leave blank)*

Publisher *(Name and complete mailing address)*

TAYLOR BALL, ELSEVIER INC.
1600 JOHN F KENNEDY BLVD. SUITE 1800
PHILADELPHIA, PA 19103-2899

Editor *(Name and complete mailing address)*

KERRY HOLLAND, ELSEVIER INC.
1600 JOHN F KENNEDY BLVD. SUITE 1800
PHILADELPHIA, PA 19103-2899

Managing Editor *(Name and complete mailing address)*

PATRICK MANLEY, ELSEVIER INC.
1600 JOHN F KENNEDY BLVD. SUITE 1800
PHILADELPHIA, PA 19103-2899

10. Owner *(Do not leave blank. If the publication is owned by a corporation, give the name and address of the corporation immediately followed by the names and addresses of all stockholders owning or holding 1 percent or more of the total amount of stock. If not owned by a corporation, give the names and addresses of the individual owners. If owned by a partnership or other unincorporated firm, give its name and address as well as those of each individual owner. If the publication is published by a nonprofit organization, give its name and address.)*

Full Name	Complete Mailing Address
WHOLLY OWNED SUBSIDIARY OF REED/ELSEVIER, US HOLDINGS	1600 JOHN F KENNEDY BLVD. SUITE 1800 PHILADELPHIA, PA 19103-2899

11. Known Bondholders, Mortgagees, and Other Security Holders Owning or Holding 1 Percent or More of Total Amount of Bonds, Mortgages, or Other Securities. If none, check box ► ☐ None

Full Name	Complete Mailing Address
N/A	

12. Tax Status *(For completion by nonprofit organizations authorized to mail at nonprofit rates) (Check one)*
The purpose, function, and nonprofit status of this organization and the exempt status for federal income tax purposes:
☒ Has Not Changed During Preceding 12 Months
☐ Has Changed During Preceding 12 Months *(Publisher must submit explanation of change with this statement)*

PS Form 3526, July 2014 [Page 1 of 4 (see instructions page 4)] PSN: 7530-01-000-9931 PRIVACY NOTICE: See our privacy policy on www.usps.com.

---

13. Publication Title	14. Issue Date for Circulation Data Below
GASTROINTESTINAL ENDOSCOPY CLINICS OF NORTH AMERICA	JULY 2019

15. Extent and Nature of Circulation		Average No. Copies Each Issue During Preceding 12 Months	No. Copies of Single Issue Published Nearest to Filing Date
a. Total Number of Copies *(Net press run)*		136	143
b. Paid Circulation *(By Mail and Outside the Mail)*	(1) Mailed Outside-County Paid Subscriptions Stated on PS Form 3541 *(include paid distribution above nominal rate, advertiser's proof copies, and exchange copies)*	53	63
	(2) Mailed In-County Paid Subscriptions Stated on PS Form 3541 *(Include paid distribution above nominal rate, advertiser's proof copies, and exchange copies)*	0	0
	(3) Paid Distribution Outside the Mails Including Sales Through Dealers and Carriers, Street Vendors, Counter Sales, and Other Paid Distribution Outside USPS®	23	28
	(4) Paid Distribution by Other Classes of Mail Through the USPS *(e.g., First-Class Mail®)*	0	0
c. Total Paid Distribution *(Sum of 15b (1), (2), (3), and (4))*	►	76	91
d. Free or Nominal Rate Distribution *(By Mail and Outside the Mail)*	(1) Free or Nominal Rate Outside-County Copies included on PS Form 3541	48	36
	(2) Free or Nominal Rate In-County Copies included on PS Form 3541	0	0
	(3) Free or Nominal Rate Copies Mailed at Other Classes Through the USPS *(e.g., First-Class Mail)*	0	0
	(4) Free or Nominal Rate Distribution Outside the Mail *(Carriers or other means)*	0	0
e. Total Free or Nominal Rate Distribution *(Sum of 15d (1), (2), (3) and (4))*	►	48	36
f. Total Distribution *(Sum of 15c and 15e)*	►	124	127
g. Copies not Distributed *(See Instructions to Publishers #4 (page #3))*	►	12	15
h. Total *(Sum of 15f and g)*	►	136	143
i. Percent Paid *(15c divided by 15f times 100)*	►	61.29%	71.65%

* If you are claiming electronic copies, go to line 16 on page 3. If you are not claiming electronic copies, skip to line 17 on page 3.

16. Electronic Copy Circulation		Average No. Copies Each Issue During Preceding 12 Months	No. Copies of Single Issue Published Nearest to Filing Date
a. Paid Electronic Copies	►		
b. Total Paid Print Copies (Line 15c) + Paid Electronic Copies (Line 16a)	►		
c. Total Print Distribution (Line 15f) + Paid Electronic Copies (Line 16a)	►		
d. Percent Paid (Both Print & Electronic Copies) (16b divided by 16c × 100)	►		

☒ I certify that 50% of all my distributed copies (electronic and print) are paid above a nominal price.

17. Publication of Statement of Ownership

☒ If the publication is a general publication, publication of this statement is required. Will be printed
in the OCTOBER 2019 issue of this publication.

☐ Publication not required.

18. Signature and Title of Editor, Publisher, Business Manager, or Owner

STEPHEN R. BUSHING - INVENTORY DISTRIBUTION CONTROL MANAGER

[signature]

Date 9/18/2019

I certify that all information furnished on this form is true and complete. I understand that anyone who furnishes false or misleading information on this form or who omits material or information requested on the form may be subject to criminal sanctions (including fines and imprisonment) and/or civil sanctions (including civil penalties).

PS Form 3526, July 2014 (Page 2 of 4) PRIVACY NOTICE: See our privacy policy on www.usps.com

Moving?

Make sure your subscription moves with you!

To notify us of your new address, find your **Clinics Account Number** (located on your mailing label above your name), and contact customer service at:

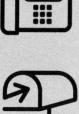

Email: journalscustomerservice-usa@elsevier.com

800-654-2452 (subscribers in the U.S. & Canada)
314-447-8871 (subscribers outside of the U.S. & Canada)

Fax number: 314-447-8029

Elsevier Health Sciences Division
Subscription Customer Service
3251 Riverport Lane
Maryland Heights, MO 63043

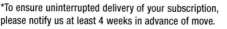

*To ensure uninterrupted delivery of your subscription, please notify us at least 4 weeks in advance of move.

ELSEVIER

Printed and bound by CPI Group (UK) Ltd, Croydon, CR0 4YY

08/05/2025

01864747-0006